About The Author

Ian Wishart is an award-winning journalist and author, with a 30 year career in radio, television and magazines, a #1 talk radio show and five #1 bestselling books to his credit. Together with his wife Heidi, they edit and publish the news magazine *Investigate* and the news website www.investigatedaily.com.

For Heidi

Vitamin D

Ian Wishart

HOWLING AT THE MOON PUBLISHING LTD

First edition published 2012
Howling At The Moon Publishing Ltd
PO Box 188, Kaukapakapa
Auckland 0843, NEW ZEALAND

www.howlingatthemoon.com
email: editorial@investigatemagazine.com
Copyright © Ian Wishart
Copyright © Howling At The Moon Publishing Ltd, 2012

ISBN 978-0-9876573-1-2

Typeset in Adobe Garamond Pro and Monotype Modern
Cover concept: Ian Wishart, Heidi Wishart, Bozidar Jokanovic
Book Design: Bozidar Jokanovic

To get another copy of this book airmailed to you anywhere in the world, or to purchase a fully text-searchable digital edition, visit our website:
WWW.HOWLINGATTHEMOON.COM

Contents

INTRODUCTION

Seven years ago, I began researching this book. I didn't know it then, of course. At the time vitamin D was an 'emerging issue' mostly confined to the medical literature and with little spillover into the popular press, particularly in Australia and New Zealand.

While the northern hemisphere was more attuned to the lack of vitamin D available at higher latitudes, the sunny south was blissfully ignorant. It wasn't possible to be vitamin D deficient down under, or so they thought.

Investigate magazine became the first mainstream media outlet in New Zealand to raise the vitamin D debate, and question whether our national obsession with slip, slop, slap was actually costing lives, not saving them.

For taking that stand, based on an ever growing body of literature, we were pilloried at the time by the establishment and by other media outlets raised on a diet of bureaucratic mushroom food.

It's funny how things change. In the last 12 months it's been hard to escape magazine and newspaper stories raising exactly the same issues we did all those years ago. Suddenly 25-hydroxyvitamin-D is the vitamin-du-jour. It's everywhere.

One thing hasn't changed, however. The health bureaucracy is still dishing out mushroom food to the news media.

Hence this book. Since 2005, I've set my inbox to receive daily Google news alerts on vitamin D studies so I could keep up with the science. Every morning, a summary of half a dozen or so of the world headlines on the subject were there to peruse, 365 days a year for seven years. That's somewhere north of 15,000 news stories and scientific studies in my files. I've interviewed key people on both sides of the debate over the years and written many feature articles and news stories.

What this book attempts to do is collate the latest cutting edge research to give you the big picture on vitamin D in regard to your own health choices.

One in three of us will die from heart disease, one in three from cancer, and Alzheimer's has a one-in-two chance of taking us if we make it to old age. Amongst the rest of us, well, the Devil will take the hindmost. In the race for a better life and a happier future, we're all seeking that miracle ingredient that will actually stack the odds in our favour.

Is vitamin D that miracle?

As parents, we are concerned not just for our own health but our children's. We spend fortunes on educational toys, extracurricular activities, anything to give our child the edge in an unforgiving world. None of us want to cause our children to be mentally or physically disadvantaged in any way.

Yet in dutifully listening to advice about avoiding the sun, in wearing make-up foundation with all-day sunscreen built in, we may have condemned not just ourselves but our children to a higher risk of some of the nastiest disorders known to humanity.

Vitamin D turns out to be the page upon which the story of life has been written.

Read the peer reviewed science in these pages and decide for yourself whether this is one supplement you need to take very seriously and, based on the evidence, frequently.

IMPORTANT NOTICE

What you are about to read is not intended as medical advice for your personal situation, because there is no such thing as a one-size-fits-all solution. Most of you reading this will be vitamin D deficient or insufficient as defined by the latest internationally-accepted standards. If you wish to begin supplementation with some of the higher doses used by doctors and scientists in this book, see your own doctor first to ensure there is no clash with existing medication or an underlying health issue.

If necessary, donate a copy of the book to your local GP and let him or her pull up the medical research listed in here that's relevant to your health condition, and tailor a programme best suited to your or your family's health needs.

Chapter 1

THE STORY OF D

"There may be more beneficial than adverse effects of moderately increased sun exposure, even for total cancer mortality"

– Dr Johan Moan, Norwegian cancer researcher, 2008

The story of vitamin D is a tale as old as life itself. Ultimately, virtually all energy available to life on this planet derives from the sun. It has beaten down on the face of the earth for around 4.5 billion years, yet life has emerged and thrived, our DNA code seemingly designed to process sunlight.

Evidence of vitamin D synthesis has been found in the fossilised remains of plankton from more than 750 million years ago. With solar radiation from a young sun powering down on everything that swam, crawled, walked or grew, life could not have survived without some kind of mechanism to use and/or deflect the unrelenting energy emissions of the nearest star.

Plants developed photosynthesis and turned sunlight

into food. Vertebrates converted sunlight into bones.

Synthesising vitamin D is crucial for developing strong skeletons. Without that process, bones remain fragile and/or soft. The mighty dinosaurs would have collapsed under their own weight into piles of flesh and lard, without vitamin D.

How then do animals cope with skin cancer? Surely staying in sunlight all day gives them a higher risk than humans? Apparently not. While skin cancers of various kinds, including melanoma, are quite common in animals, they are rarely fatal and can often be left untreated, say vets.[1] Animal bodies are sufficiently acclimatised to radiation to be able to keep skin cancers mostly under control. Natural selection works to ensure that tougher gene lines survive and the weaker ones are weeded out.

In apes, the mechanism for utilising vitamin D is different from humans. When solar radiation hits an ape or monkey, the vitamin D is created in the skin, but then secreted back up into the fur. It is from licking themselves while grooming, or picking out bugs from the fur, that the vitamin D gets into the mouth and is digested. It is from there that primates utilise vitamin D for bone and general health.

So what went wrong with humans?

---

1   "Gray area" by Ken Marcella, D.V.M,
http://www.horses-and-horse-information.com/
articles/0701melanoma.shtml

For tens of thousands of years we have adapted to solar radiation, the most obvious example being racial skin colouring. Humans living near the tropics are darker skinned thanks to melanin, the protective pigment in our cells that is switched on by sunlight as a defence mechanism against UV radiation. Populations living further north or south of the equator developed lighter skins, but why?

It now turns out that darker skins in the higher latitudes don't allow enough vitamin D into your body because they block the weaker sun more efficiently. Darker-skinned people in Europe and North America, or New Zealand and southern Australia, for example, have greater health problems than light-skinned people. It is only in the past decade, however, that we have really become aware of just why that is: a lack of vitamin D.

The first records we can examine, with hindsight, for clues, date back to 450 BC, when Greek historian Herodotus noted that warriors from Persia had soft skulls. Nowadays, we know this to be a bone condition called osteomalacia, the adult form of "rickets". Herodotus reckoned the Persians had soft heads because they wore turbans. Hippocrates, from whom medicine derives its 'Hippocratic oath', wrote about rickets around the same time, and also prescribed sunlight as a treatment for tuberculosis – a disease now known to be affected by vitamin D.

No one back then knew, of course, about the existence of vitamin D as such, or the precise reactions that sunlight triggered in the human body.

It wasn't until the dawning of the age of modern science that researchers began making a closer connection between some of these conditions. In 1789, for example, a doctor prescribed cod-liver oil – now known as an excellent food source of vitamin D – for chronic rheumatism. Cod-liver oil was then experimented with, successfully, as a treatment for children with rickets in the 1820s. But it wasn't for a further 100 years that science could finally put a name to the mysterious vitamin itself. Two lines of research, one working with cod-liver oil and another with sunlight, converged in the 1930s with the discovery that sunlight was creating in skin the same substance found in cod-liver oil. They called it vitamin D, and it formed when the substance 7-Dehydrocholesterol was exposed to ultraviolet radiation.[2]

For decades, science has known about vitamin D being crucial to bone and skeletal health, and children in the forties and fifties were routinely given doses of cod-liver oil and sunlight for good health.

During the same period, however, sunscreens were

---

2   There are two primary forms of vitamin D. Ergocalciferol, known as vitamin D2, is obtained from food sources. Cholecalciferol, or vitamin D3, is produced when sunlight strikes your skin and converts cholesterol to a fat-soluble compound.

beginning to capture the public imagination and of course industrialisation was keeping people working behind closed doors in dark offices and factories.

Society was changing. For the first time in thousands of years, it was possible for people to really protect themselves from the sun's UV radiation. Yet at the same time, skin cancer cases suddenly began to escalate.

In the early 1990s, a Norwegian Cancer Institute research scientist, Professor Johan Moan, made a significant announcement in the *British Journal of Cancer*: while the annual incidence of melanoma in Norway had quadrupled between 1957 and 1984, there had been no corresponding change in the ozone layer over the region. "Ozone depletion is not the cause of the increase in skin cancers," his medical journal report notes.

As if to emphasise the rapid increase in skin cancer rates, the Norwegians re-analysed the data just a few years later and found the rates had grown again, a 600% increase in skin cancer between 1960 and 1990 – just thirty years! Yet still no change in ozone levels.

Why was skin cancer rising when supposedly increased UV through the ozone hole was not actually causing it?

For a long while, research on vitamin D languished on the fringes. The primary area of interest to public health authorities was putting in place campaigns easily understood by the public in order to reduce the growing epidemic of skin cancer.

Slip, slop, slap became a global catchphrase.

By the mid 2000s, however, strange results were emerging from scientific studies. Time after time, people with low vitamin D levels were found to have a higher risk of dying from cancer or heart disease.

In January 2008, Norway's Johan Moan was back at centre stage with the publication of a report in America's *Proceedings of the National Academy of Sciences* journal,[3] based on new cancer data from New Zealand, Australia and Scandinavia. Moan had chosen the antipodes because the two southern hemisphere nations have the highest skin cancer rates and strongest UV radiation in the world, thanks largely to the ozone hole over Antarctica during the southern summer and the current tilt of earth's axis.

Moan wanted to compare skin cancer data from New Zealand and Australia, with the same statistics in the Northern Hemisphere. His team chose racial and skin types that are closely related genetically, in order to get the best possible comparison. What they found shook up the world of vitamin D research.

While people downunder suffer much higher melanoma rates than their colleagues in the north, Australia and New Zealand's survival rates are – paradoxically

---

3   "Addressing the health benefits and risks, involving vitamin D or skin cancer, of increased sun exposure," Moan et al, Proceedings of the National Academy of Sciences, *PNAS January 15, 2008 vol. 105 no. 2 668-673.* http://www.pnas.org/content/105/2/668.long

– much higher on a victim-for-victim comparison. The same applies to internal cancers like breast, prostate or colon – although Australasia suffers higher rates of those cancers, residents of New Zealand and Oz are also more likely to survive them.

Australians, who get more sun than kiwis, are more likely to survive their cancers than New Zealanders are, lending further weight to the theory.

What remains up in the air is the exact cause of many of these cancers. Modern diets are full of agricultural chemicals, with one Spanish study published 2008 finding every single Spanish citizen (100% of the study sample) has one or more agricultural pesticides circulating in their blood at significant levels. New Zealand and Australia, as heavy agricultural producers, may have correspondingly higher cancer rates for that reason. Even so, sunlight appears to have a significant impact in helping survive those cancers.

The data mined for the PNAS study raised doubts about whether sunlight was the driving cause of melanoma.

"The main arguments against the concept that sun exposure causes cutaneous malignant melanoma (CMM) are that: 1) CMM is more common among persons with indoor work than among those people with outdoor work; 2) in younger generations, more CMMs arise per unit skin area on partly shielded areas (trunk and legs) than on face and neck; and 3) CMMs sometimes arise on totally shielded areas [soles of feet, palms, inside the eyeball]."

Nonetheless, the PNAS study suggests that a "significant fraction" of malignant melanomas may be caused by sun exposure.

Leaving aside the cause, however, the PNAS study had some breakthrough data on cancer survival rates. If your vitamin D levels are high, you are around 30% more likely to survive "prostate, breast, colon and lung cancers, as well as lymphomas and even melanomas," reports the study.

"Other investigators have found comparable results. These data argue for a positive role of sun-induced vitamin D in cancer prognosis, or that a good vitamin D status is advantageous when in combination with standard cancer therapies."

At the stage the research was done, the upper "safe limit" of vitamin D supplement intake was believed by regulators to be 200 international units a day. Whilst the human body had become supremely efficient at converting sunlight to vitamin D without any toxic effects, too much vitamin D in food had been shown to be harmful in the past.

Moan's study raised a conundrum, because it found the levels of vitamin D needed in the blood to help protect against cancer were far higher than you could achieve in 2008 taking the maximum recommended supplement of 200 IU a day in pill form. The only option then, appeared to be sunlight as a source of healthy vitamin D, which put Moan directly in the firing line of the skin cancer research community. That didn't stop Moan from stating the obvious:

"Thus we conclude that…the sun is an important source of vitamin D…So far, epidemiological data for cancer argue for an overall positive role of sun-induced vitamin D. There may be more beneficial than adverse effects of moderately increased sun exposure, even for total cancer mortality."

To understand why this might be the case, you first need to understand a little about vitamin D. Ignore some of the long words and just follow the ball in the brief description that follows.

When UVB rays from the sun strike our skin, they set off a chemical reaction pre-programmed into our DNA. Dermatologists call the process "DNA damage" in a bid to scare people, but it's entirely natural and has been part of our life cycle since the very beginning of humanity. The chemical in the skin that reacts to sunlight is called 7-dehydro-cholesterol which, as its name suggests, is a type of cholesterol. Without it, the reaction could not happen.

The 7-dehydro-cholesterol is transformed by the UV and thermal energy into the chemical we call vitamin D3, or cholecalciferol. This chemical is then circulated through the bloodstream into the liver where it is "hydroxylated" into 25(OH)D (aka calcidiol) – the actual variant of vitamin D that's measured in blood serum levels.

Still watching the ball? The 25(OH)D is then spun off by the kidney and converted into a further form known as $1,25(OH)_2D$, (calcitriol) which is the variant used to regulate calcium absorption in your body and perform a whole lot of previously unknown functions.

"$1,25(OH)_2D$ acts as a molecular switch," writes vitamin D researcher John Cannell, activating "target genes" and receptors throughout the body. One of the recent discoveries, for example, is that our immune systems use it to manufacture "naturally-occurring human antibiotics" within our bodies. If you have low vitamin D, your body's immune system can't manufacture its own antibiotics, and the implications of that don't require a rocket science degree.[4]

But here's the twist. Up until only a few years ago, it was assumed $1,25(OH)_2D$ could only be manufactured by the kidneys, and only for the purposes of the well understood skeletal health system. Instead, most organs of the body have since been discovered to have the ability to generate $1,25(OH)_2D$ for their own purposes. The brain, the heart, the stomach, the lungs, just some of the previously unknown systems for processing vitamin D independent of the kidneys. No other vitamin is like it.

---

4   "Diagnosis and treatment of vitamin D deficiency", Cannell et al, *Journal of Expert Opinion in Pharmacotherapy, 2008, 9(1):1-12*

The argument that vitamin D had special powers gained weight from another study, a randomised controlled trial of vitamin D over a four year period, which found a dramatic decrease in cancers amongst those who were given 1,110 IU (international units) of vitamin D3 each day, compared to those on a placebo.

The study followed 403 women from Nebraska, and measured them against a control group of 206 on placebo. After the trial, the vitamin D users had 77% fewer cancers than placebo users.[5]

While the debate about supplementation vs sunbathing, or even a combination of both, is ongoing, the message that vitamin D appears to lower cancer risk is clear.

Of course, as with all things, there is a trade-off between increasing sun exposure for your family's health, and increasing the risk of skin cancer. But the numbers tell the story: In 2004, 7,900 Americans died of melanoma. On the flip side of that coin and using the above data, 45,000 Americans are believed to have died from cancers that they could have survived or avoided with greater exposure to the sun. In other words, you may be nine times more likely to die from cancer caused or aggravated by a *lack* of sunlight, than you are from skin cancer caused by sunlight.

---

5   "Vitamin D and calcium supplementation reduces cancer risk," Lappe et al, *American Journal of Clinical Nutrition*, 2007, 85(6):1586-91

A 2009 report delivered to the Canadian government estimated that if vitamin D levels were increased across the board, 37,000 fewer people would die prematurely in Canada each year as a result of avoidable disease, saving taxpayers some $14 billion annually and saving an enormous amount of family grief.[6]

Yet the extent of vitamin D deficiency is actually huge. A telltale sign is the huge rise in the number of cases of rickets – a disease thought vanquished in the early 20th century – across the world. Characterised by bone deformities, children and babies can also suffer seizures. Hospital emergency departments in London, New York, Sydney and Auckland are routinely seeing children with rickets now.

Low vitamin D levels are the cause. A study of inpatients at Boston's Massachusetts General Hospital found 57% had vitamin D levels in the blood that were deficient.[7] Thirty one percent of Australians are in the same boat.[8] Even in Melbourne and Adelaide at

---

6 "An estimate of the economic burden and premature deaths due to vitamin D deficiency in Canada," Grant et al, *Mol. Nutr. Food Res.* 2010, *54*, 1172–1181, http://www.vitamindsociety.org/pdf/ Grant%202010%20-%20vitamin%20D%20deficiency%20in%20 Canada.pdf

7 "Diagnosis and treatment of vitamin D deficiency," Cannell et al, *Expert Opinion in Pharmacotherapy*, 2008 9(1), citing "Hypovitaminosis D in medical inpatients," Thomas et al, *New England Journal of Medicine*, 1998; 338(12):777-83

8 "Prevalence of vitamin D deficiency and its determinants in Australian adults etc," Daly et al, *Oxford Journal of Clinical*

the end of summer, 42% of women and 27% of men were vitamin D deficient. Given the Aussie summer sun, they shouldn't have been.

As vitamin D researcher Cedric Garland announced to the world, getting people to spend 15 minutes a day in the sun without sunscreen could save ten lives from cancer alone, for every extra skin cancer death caused by increased sun exposure.

It was this kind of information that caused doctors the world over to sit up and think: was the message on staying sun-safe the wrong message? Had the pendulum of caution swung too far, to the point where it was causing more cancers in other areas? What exactly was the link between vitamin D and cancer mortality? Why was melanoma not nearly as fatal in New Zealand and Australia, despite the strongest UV radiation in the world?

Could it be that the sunshine vitamin held secrets essential to life, secrets only now being unlocked?

Endocrinology, 2012 Jul; 77(1):26-35

Chapter 2

ALZHEIMER'S CURSE

"We hypothesize that good vitamin D levels might prevent or mitigate the disease"

– Associate Professor of Geriatrics Robert Przybelski, 2007

One of the early studies to show promise involved the mental deterioration of Alzheimer's. It's a shocking, debilitating disease, for which no cure exists. Once diagnosed, sufferers are usually dead after seven years, and only little more than two percent are alive by 14 years.

Around one in fifty people aged up to 64 suffer Alzheimer's, jumping to around one in five people between the ages of 75 and 84, and nearly one in two people aged 85 and over. In other words, if you managed to rack up your allotted three-score years and ten, there's nearly a fifty-fifty chance Alzheimer's will come for you.

The disease degenerates your mind, starting slowly with a little bit of fuzziness around the edges, then gradually robbing you of short and medium term memory until you reach the final stages where you are talking with fairies, dribbling from both sides of your mouth and needing around the clock nursing and toilet care.

The spectre of Alzheimer's haunts Baby Boomers and Gen-Xers so much that its one of the driving forces behind pleas to introduce voluntary euthanasia. "Kill me if I get Alzheimer's," they beg. Well, there might be a better option.

When a small observational study by University of Wisconsin researchers was published online in January 2007 showing a significant association for the first time between low levels of vitamin D in the blood of Alzheimer's patients and poor performance on a cognitive test, people's ears pricked up.

The study was prompted after family members of the Alzheimer's patients reported how well they were performing and acting within weeks of being put on large doses of prescription vitamin D, said lead author Robert Przybelski, an associate professor of geriatric medicine at the University of Wisconsin.

"We hypothesize that good vitamin D levels might prevent or mitigate the disease," Przybelski said.[9]

The study noted that neurons, like many other cells,

9   "Is vitamin D important for preserving cognition? A positive correlation of serum 25-hydroxyvitamin D concentration with cognitive function," Przybelski RJ, Binkley NC, *Archives of Biochemistry & Biophysics*, 2007 Apr 15;460(2):202-5. Epub 2007 Jan 8

have vitamin D receptors. It says vitamin D might enhance levels of important brain chemicals and that it also might help protect brain cells.

That was 2007. Rapidly, researchers moved into overdrive. Could vitamin D not only improve the minds of Alzheimer's sufferers, but perhaps even help stave it off?

A Boston based study published 2008 examined more than a thousand "elders" – people aged 65 to 99 – for their performance in cognitive mental function tests, relative to their vitamin D blood serum levels.

To understand a lot of the research presented in this book, you'll need to become familiar with different scientific descriptions of the same thing. In this case, blood serum of vitamin D, usually grouped under the name "25(OH)D", is measured relative to its volume in blood.

So far, so good. The scientists however use two different measuring systems and you will find different studies use one or the other. One is expressed as nanograms per millilitre, or "ng/ml". The other rival way of expressing this is nanomoles per litre, "nmol/L", but the numbers are not identical. Multiply ng by 2.5 and you'll get the nmol figure. For rule of thumb purposes, I've set out below the two different scales of blood serum vitamin D measurement. Come back to this conversion chart for further reference if you need to:[10]

10   "Ideal Level" is recommended by the Vitamin D Council.

Ideal Vitamin D Level	Insufficient Level[11]	Deficient Level	Seriously Deficient Level
125 – 200 nmol/L	<75 nmol/L	<50 nmol/L	<25 nmol/L
50 – 80 ng/ml	<30 ng/ml	<20 ng/ml	<10 ng/ml

It's worth noting that 50 ng/ml is the natural blood level of vitamin D often found in people who've worked outside over summer, as humans have done for millennia. Armed with that, we return to the Boston study.

Sixty-five percent of the "elders" had 25(OH)D levels below 50 nmol/L, putting them into the seriously insufficient category. Eighteen percent were listed as deficient, with less than 25 nmol/L.

Adjustments in the analysis were made for age, sex, race, body mass index, education, residence area, kidney function, seasonality, physical activity, and alcohol use. Even after all that, the elders with higher vitamin D levels scored significantly higher in tests including "trails… digit symbol…matrix reasoning…block design".

The analysts dug deeper, adjusting for possible interference from other hormones in the system, B vitamins or multivitamin use. Despite all of that, people with the highest levels of vitamin D still emerged the winners.[12]

The remaining levels are those defined by health agencies. Many agencies are now beginning to realise "deficiency" may actually set in where "insufficiency" currently sits. This will become obvious to you as you read some of the study results.

11   The abbreviation ≤ represents "less than or equal to", for those who have long forgotten the intricacies of school maths. The opposite is 'greater than'.

12   "Vitamin D Is Associated With Cognitive Function in

A European study of healthy men aged 40+ found a similar link between low vitamin D levels and slower mental skills.

"In this population-based study of European men aged ≥ 40 years we observed a significant, independent association between a slower information processing speed (as assessed by the DSST test) and lower levels of 25(OH)D. The association appeared strongest among those with a 25(OH)D level less than ~35 nmol/L.[13]

"Although the magnitude of the association between 25(OH)D and processing speed was comparatively small, if cognitive function can be improved by a simple intervention such as vitamin D supplementation, this would have potentially important implications for population health."

In other words, if you want to keep your wits about you, vitamin D is crucial.

A 2011 study in Turkey of 125 geriatric patients found elderly people who took summer walks in the sun were 73% more capable of scoring highly in cognitive tests.[14]

Elders Receiving Home Health Services," Buell et al, *Journals of Gerontology*, J Gerontol A Biol Sci Med Sci (2009) 64A (8): 888-895. doi: 10.1093/gerona/glp0

13   "Association Between 25-Hydroxyvitamin D Levels And Cognitive Performance In Middle-Aged And Older European Men," Lee et al, *Journal of Neurology, Neurosurgery & Psychiatry 80*, 7 (2009) 722

14   "Predictors of clock drawing test (CDT) performance in elderly patients attending an internal medicine outpatient clinic: A pilot study on sun exposure and physical activity", Aydin et al,

By May 2011, researchers had well and truly realised they were onto something.

"There is evidence that the vast majority of hospitalised patients have vitamin D deficiency. Vitamin D deficiency is a poorly-recognised pandemic..."[15]

A lack of vitamin D, they warned, was turning out to be one of the biggest canaries in the mineshaft in the entire health system.

What scientists had found is that the human body is full of what we now know are "vitamin D receptors", or VDRs. These are docking bays where the body is designed to receive vitamin D, docking bays which for the last century we'd evidently forgotten how to use. The less of the vitamin we obtained, the more our bodies began to break down, and the greater the cost of treating us in the health system.

The benefits of vitamin D as listed by Youssef and his team included "antimicrobial and immunomodulation effects", which is geek-speak for germ-killing and immune system stimulation, "as well as benefits on cardiovascular health, autoimmune disease, cancer and metabolism. Vitamin D deficiency increases mortality [kills you sooner] and even a modest amount of

Archives of Gerontology and Geriatrics, Volume 52, Issue 3, May–June 2011, Pages e226–e231

15   "Vitamin D deficiency: implications for acute care in the elderly and in patients with chronic illness," Youssef et al, _Geriatrics & Gerontology International_, Vol 11, issue 4, Oct 2011:395-407

vitamin D may enhance longevity."

In a study published March 2012, the health files of 498 elderly women were examined in the French city of Toulouse, to determine whether their vitamin D status was an accurate predictor of how quickly they would succumb to Alzheimer's Disease or, as they described it, "an independent predictor of the onset of dementia within seven years among women aged 75 years and older."[16]

The sample group was assessed at the end of seven years and split into three: those with no dementia; those with Alzheimer's Disease; those with other dementias. They had all been tested and questioned at the start of the seven year trial, and their scores (described in the literature as "baseline results") noted down.

Of the nearly 500 women, 70 were Alzheimer's sufferers by the end of it, and that group had the lowest vitamin D levels.

The twenty percent of women who had the highest vitamin D levels had a 77% lower risk of developing Alzheimer's during the seven years, compared with the 80% of women with lower vitamin D, leading to an inescapable study conclusion: "Higher vitamin D dietary intake was associated with a lower risk of

16   "Higher Vitamin D dietary intake is associated with lower risk of Alzheimer's Disease: a 7-year follow-up," Annweiler et al, *Journals of Gerontology*, first published online April 13, 2012, doi: 10.1093/Gerona/gls107

developing Alzheimer's Disease among older women".

Attention has turned to "how" and "why" questions. What is it about vitamin D that assists in warding off one of the most dreaded incurable disorders known to man? In April 2012 a British team from the University of Exeter reported:[17]

"The role of vitamin D in skeletal health is well established, but more recent findings have also linked vitamin D deficiency to a range of non-skeletal conditions such as cardiovascular disease, cancer, stroke and metabolic disorders including diabetes.

"Cognitive impairment and dementia must now be added to this list. Vitamin D receptors [VDRs] are widespread in brain tissue, and vitamin D's biologically active form, $1,25(OH)_2D3$, has shown protective effects including the clearance of amyloid plaques, a hallmark of Alzheimer's Disease."

Noting that "the risk of cognitive impairment" was "four times greater" in people with vitamin D levels below 25 nmol/L, when compared with those at minimum adequate levels of 75 nmol/L, the study's lead author Maya Soni goes on to link vitamin D's effect on dementia with the seemingly related fact that people with low levels are also more likely to suffer serious brain bleeds "and fatal stroke".

---

17   "Vitamin D and cognitive function," Soni et al, *Scandinavian Journal of Clinical and Laboratory Investigation*, April 2012, Vol. 72, No. S243:79-82

It is the "clearance of amyloid plaques, a hallmark of Alzheimer's", that is now one of the focal points for researchers. The next paragraph is slightly technical, but given your odds of developing Alzheimer's down the track and turning into a household vegetable, what follows could be very important to you.

A just published study in the *Journal of Alzheimer's* reports that vitamin D is able to not just neutralise, but to actually "recover" damaged brain function:

"Brain clearance of amyloid-ß (A ß42) by innate immune cells is necessary for normal brain function. Phagocytosis [eating of] soluble A ß42 by Alzheimer's Disease (AD) macrophages is defective, recovered in all 'Type I and Type II' AD patients by 1∂,25(OH)2-vitamin D3 (1,25D3) and blocked by the nuclear vitamin D receptor [VDR]..."[18]

I could go on, but clearly you get the picture: "The structure-function results provide evidence that 1,25D3 activation of VDR-dependent genomic and non-genomic signalling, work in concert to recover dysregulated innate immune function in Alzheimer's Disease."

Another study has found that a genetic fault in one of the brain's key vitamin D receptors is associated with a higher risk of developing Alzheimer's. "We provide both statistical evidence and functional data suggesting

---

18 "Genomic and nongenomic signalling induced by 1ℓ,25(OH)2-vitamin D3 promotes the recovery of Amyloid-ß etc," Mizwicki et al, *Journal of Alzheimer's Disease*, Vol. 29, Issue 1 2012:51-62

VDR confers genetic risk for AD. Our findings are consistent with epidemiology studies suggesting that vitamin D insufficiency increases the risk of developing Alzheimer's Disease."[19]

If you want to keep your mental clock ticking, then, and lower your risks of Alzheimer's in years to come, it appears vitamin D may be the ingredient you need. But it's not just the middle-aged or elderly at risk from a vitamin D deficiency.

19   "Vitamin D receptor and Alzheimer's Disease: a genetic and functional study," Wang et al, *Neurobiology of Aging*, Vol. 33, Issue 8:1844e1-1844e9, August 2012

Chapter 3

AUTISTIC SPECTRUM DISORDERS

"The apparent increase in the prevalence of autism over the last 20 years corresponds with increasing medical advice to avoid the sun"

– Dr John Cannell, Vitamin D Council, 2008

Twenty-five years ago, your chance of giving birth to an autistic-spectrum child was somewhere north of 1:1800. Today, it's as low as 1:60. For a long time, researchers suspected the culprit was vaccination, and in particular the Measles, Mumps, Rubella (MMR) vaccine introduced for worldwide use in the 1980s. Further studies, however, have failed to find a conclusive link to the vaccine.

Something, however, must have happened to generate a rapidly rising autism rate over that time, and that 'something' must be common to our wider civilisation, like vaccination. Or maybe slip, slop, slap.

"The apparent increase in the prevalence of autism over the last 20 years corresponds with increasing medical advice to avoid the sun," wrote California doctor and psychiatrist John Cannell in a 2008 study,[20] "advice that has probably lowered vitamin D levels and would theoretically greatly lower activated vitamin D (calcitriol) levels in developing brains.

"Animal data has repeatedly shown that severe vitamin D deficiency during gestation dysregulates dozens of proteins involved in brain development and leads to rat pups with increased brain size and enlarged ventricles, abnormalities similar to those found in autistic children.

"Children with vitamin D deficient rickets have several autistic markers that apparently disappear with high-dose vitamin D treatment."

Like the Alzheimer's study in the previous chapter, Cannell's work shook up the autism world. Across the western world, sun avoidance has been one of if not *the* primary dominant public health messages of the past two decades. While correlation does not automatically prove causation, it is undeniable that the rapid take-up of the sun avoidance message, particularly by women of child-bearing age, coincides with the rapid rise of autism.

The hypothesis was simple: could a lack of vitamin D exposure in pregnancy deprive a baby's developing brain of crucial input into its VDR receptors? For

20   "Autism and vitamin D," Cannell J, *Med Hypotheses.* 2008;70(4):750-9. Epub 2007 Oct 24.

researchers, there was growing circumstantial evidence that this might be exactly the case.

Firstly, they found autism levels were considerably lower in populations who consumed high levels of oily fish – a well recognised vitamin D source – in their usual diets. In Manhattan, London, Toronto, Sydney or Auckland, oily fish is not a regular menu item for families, but in many wilder parts of the world it is.

"Consumption of vitamin D-containing fish during pregnancy reduces autistic symptoms in offspring," notes Cannell.

"Surprisingly, high maternal seafood consumption, of the type known to be contaminated with mercury, has been associated with fewer, not more, autistic markers in the offspring. Lower maternal seafood intake during pregnancy was associated with low verbal intelligence quotient, suboptimum outcomes for pro-social behaviour, fine motor, communication and social development scores.

"While the omega-3 and mercury content of fish is well known," explains Cannell, "less well known is the fact that fish is one of the few foods with significant amounts of vitamin D, which…protects the genome from damage by toxins."[21]

But there were more clues. Autism is more prevalent

---

21   "On the aetiology of autism," John Cannell, *Acta Paediatrica* 2010; 99, Issue 8:1128-1130, http://onlinelibrary.wiley.com/ doi/10.1111/j.1651-2227.2010.01883.x/full

the further north or south of the tropics that you go. It's more common in urban areas, or those with cloudier skies. In short, the distribution of autism across the planet seems to match the patterns of cancer alluded to in the first chapter and themselves now believed to be vitamin D related.

Vitamin D health problems are more common in dark-skinned people because their vitamin D levels are lower in the weaker sun of the temperate regions. Guess what? "Autism is more common in dark-skinned persons," says Cannell, who reached a shocking conclusion about what's causing autism:

"Widespread gestational and/or early childhood vitamin D deficiency may explain both the genetics and epidemiology [prevalence and spread] of autism. If so, much of the disease is iatrogenic [caused by the medical profession], brought on by medical advice to avoid the sun."

Cannell theorises that autistic children probably have a genetic pre-disposition making them vulnerable to the disorder (a bit like the faulty gene allele recently located in Alzheimer's), which is triggered by environmental events, including a lack of vitamin D. Maybe vitamin D is the crucial brick in the brain's wall that's missing; an infant's brain VDRs wait for an influx of vitamin D that never comes, and therefore the final chemical reaction, the key in the lock, to make their brains safe from the risk of autism never takes place.

This, he says, would explain the partially inherited side of autism.

Vitamin D deficiency, says Cannell, is a prime risk factor for neurodevelopmental disorders because vitamin D is a hormone that:

- Functions as a neurosteroid
- Is a potent up-regulator of nerve growth factor
- Is found in a wide variety of brain tissue very early in embryogenesis
- Offers neuroprotection, anti-epileptic effects, and immunomodulation [control of the immune system]

But what about the fact that many mothers worldwide take a daily pregnancy multi-vitamin that includes vitamin D? Surely that proves the mothers and babies should have been getting enough?

For much of the past three decades, the official recommended daily intake of vitamin D has been only 200 IU (international units) a day. In fact, this is still the current RDI recommendation for children in New Zealand today. This figure is described as "adequate" by the Cancer Society and the Ministry of Health.[22]

Yet in a controlled randomised double blind trial involving autistic children, a daily dose of 300IU still didn't get their blood serum levels anywhere close

22   See page 13 of the 2008 Cancer Society of NZ/MoH *Position Statement*

to adequate, leaving the study authors to comment: "It appears that much higher levels of vitamin D are needed to affect blood levels of vitamin D."[23]

At the risk of labouring the point, if health authorities are so far behind the eight ball in understanding vitamin D deficiency and don't even realise how much vitamin D the public actually need, can the public rely on their assurances? And to answer the question a moment ago, if pregnancy supplements for most of the past two decades have only included a few hundred units of vitamin D, mothers may as well have been 'peeing in the wind' for all the good it was doing.

John Cannell makes the same point, contrasting the tiny amounts of vitamin D in pregnancy supplements (the artificial option) with the amounts generated when a pregnant woman sunbathes (the natural option throughout history):

"Large populations of pregnant women putting small amounts of vitamin D in their mouths – in the form of prenatal vitamins – instead of generating large amounts in their skins, is novel to human brain development."

In other words, it's an experiment that's never been tried before.

"The skin's production of vitamin D is remarkably rapid and extraordinarily robust, easily exceeding rec-

23   "Effect of a vitamin/mineral supplement on children and adults with autism," Adams et al, *BMC Pediatrics* 2011, 11:111, http://www.biomedcentral.com/1471-2431/11/111

ognised dietary sources by an order of magnitude. When fair-skinned adults sunbathe in the summer for 20 minutes, they input about 20,000 IU of vitamin D to their systemic circulation within 24 hours."

Even when the D supplement in pregnancy multivitamins was boosted to 400IU, Cannell was scornful:[24]

"A 2008 review detailed the devastating effect gestational vitamin D deficiency has on developing mammalian brains. Unfortunately the tiny 10 µg (400IU) dose in prenatal vitamins is virtually irrelevant in preventing the current epidemic of gestational vitamin D deficiency.[25] For this reason, in 2007, the Canadian Paediatric Society cautioned pregnant women they may require not 400IU/day but 2000IU/day, or more, to prevent gestational vitamin D deficiency."[26]

Since Cannell first published his suspicions that the slip, slop, slap campaign may be directly responsible for autism, the evidence has poured in to back up those suspicions.

A study in California found pregnant women whose

---

24   "On the aetiology of autism," John Cannell, *Acta Paediatrica* 2010; 99, Issue 8:1128-1130, http://onlinelibrary.wiley.com/ doi/10.1111/j.1651-2227.2010.01883.x/full

25   "Vitamin D deficiency and insufficiency in pregnant women: a longitudinal study," Holmes et al, *British Journal of Nutrition*, 2009; 31:1-6

26   "Vitamin D supplementation: recommendations for Canadian mothers and infants," Canadian Paediatric Society, *Journal of Paediatric Child Health*, 2007; 12:583-98

first trimester fell in the winter months were at a higher risk of having an autistic child.[27]

In Sweden, immigrant mothers from Somalia have been the subjects of two major studies recently. One found that black Somalian mothers are 630% more likely than white Swedes to give birth in Sweden to an autistic child, and dark-skinned mothers from East Asia were the next highest risk group at 240%,[28] while the second study found black African mothers were five times more likely to have autistic children. In all cases, the Somali mothers had much lower vitamin D levels, and 80% of their affected children had some kind of attention-deficit hyperactivity disorder.[29]

That hyperactivity link alerted the researchers, who found that rats deprived of vitamin D during brain development become hyperactive.[30]

That news alone raises questions about whether ADHD's explosion over the past twenty years is also slip, slop, slap related.

A third study, examining the rates of autism in dark-

27   "Month of conception and risk of autism," Zerbo et al, *Epidemiology*, July 2011, Vol 22, Issue 4:469-475

28   "Risk factors for autism and Asperger syndrome," Haglund, N, and Kallen, K, *Autism*, March 2011, vol 15 no. 2:163-183

29   "Prevalence of autism in children of Somali origin living in Stockholm," Barnevik-Olsson et al, *Developmental Medicine & Child Neurology*, Dec 2010, Vol 52, Issue 12:1167-1168

30   "Hyperlocomotion associated with transient prenatal vitamin D deficiency etc," Burne et al, *Behav. Brain Res*, 2006; 174:119-24

skinned immigrant mothers, found a "highly significant" link between black ethnicity and autism. "The risk was also very significant for autism associated with mental retardation. These results are consistent with the maternal vitamin D insufficiency hypothesis."[31]

The study called for urgent randomised, controlled trials to document "the effect of maternal vitamin D insufficiency during pregnancy on the foetal brain and the window of vulnerability. This review stresses the importance of monitoring vitamin D levels in pregnant women, especially those who are immigrant, dark-skinned or veiled."

However, Somali migrants in Europe are not the only ones suddenly giving birth to autistic children.

"Three of four recent US studies found a higher incidence of autism in black children, sometimes appreciably higher," John Cannell revealed. "As Fernell et al report, the Somali immigrants in Sweden call autism 'the Swedish disease', and Somali immigrants in Minnesota call it 'the American disease', but in equatorial Somalia, autism has no name."[32]

The Somali community's autism webpage in the United States carries a poignant front page support message from down under:

---

31   "Prevalence of autism according to maternal immigrant status and ethnic origin," Dealberto, M J, *Acta Psychiatrica Scandinavia*, May 2011, Vol. 123, Issue 5:339-348

32   "On the aetiology of autism," John J Cannell, *Acta Paediatrica*, May 2010 " http://www.ncbi.nlm.nih.gov/pmc/articles/PMC2913107/pdf/apa0099-1128.pdf

"I just saw your website and wanted to thank you. I am a Somali social worker in New Zealand and see lots of Somali kids born here that also have autism. Thanks for being brave in the eyes of so many."[33]

Remember, the central premise is simple: dark-skinned people are designed to live under tropical sun, and their skins are too dark to process enough vitamin D in colder climates, especially when religious or cultural veils are added to the mix.[34]

Adding weight to the vitamin D theory, a study of the prevalence of autism in sunny Oman, in Arabia, found 1 case per 7,000 children. Not one in 60.[35] In sunny Israel, the incidence is reportedly 1 in 5,000.[36] Interestingly, before the sun avoidance campaigns took hold from the eighties onwards, Israel's diagnosed autism cases were as low as one in half a million. In cold, northern Japan on

33   Somali American Autism Support, http://saaswa.org/?page_id=94 accessed July 2012

34   A study of Masai tribesmen in eastern Africa found their vitamin D levels were a staggering 47.6 ng/ml (119 nmol/L) on average, more than double the average of Africans living in America. See "Traditionally living populations in East Africa have a mean serum 25-hydroxyvitamin D concentration of 115 nmol/L," Luxwolda et al. *British Journal of Nutrition*. 2012. doi:10.1017/S0007114511007161

35   "Brief report: prevalence of autistic spectrum disorders in the Sultanate of Oman," Yahya et al, *Journal of Autism and Developmental Disorders*, 2011, Vol. 41, Issue 6:821-825

36   "Time trends in reported autistic spectrum disorders in Israel, 1972-2004," Senecky et al, *Israeli Medical Assn Journal*, 2009 Jan;11(1):30-3 http://www.ima.org.il/imaj/ar09jan-05.pdf

the other hand, one in 62 children in Yokohama were found to be suffering from autistic spectrum disorder.[37]

"Another of the mysteries of autism," says Cannell, "is the apparent increased incidence of autism in the children of richer, college-educated parents, especially women.

"If the vitamin D theory is true, autism should be more common in richer, well-educated mothers, who are more likely than other mothers to practice sun-avoidance and use sunblock."

Sure enough, that's exactly what researchers have found.[38]

Study after study is now drawing a direct link between mothers who follow sunsmart advice, and a much higher risk of having autistic babies, such as this one from 2012:

"Vitamin D deficiency – either during pregnancy or early childhood – may be an environmental trigger for ASD (autistic spectrum disorder) in individuals genetically predisposed for the broad phenotype of autism. On the basis of the results of the present review, we argue for the recognition of this possibly important role of vitamin

---

37   "No effect of MMR withdrawal on the incidence of autism: a total population study," Honda et al, *Journal of Child Psychology and Psychiatry*, Volume 46, Issue 6, pages 572–579, June 2005
38   "Sociodemographic risk factors for autism in a US metropolitan area," Bhasin TK, Schendel D, *Journal of Autism and Developmental Disorders*, 2007; 37:667-77. See also "Geographic distribution of autism in California," Van Meter et al, *Autism Research*, 2010; 3:19-29

D in ASD, and for urgent research in the field."[39]

Or:

"The increasing incidence of vitamin D insufficiency is likely also associated with the increased risk of autism spectrum disorders as reported in this cohort, thus supporting the hypothesis that gestational vitamin D deficiency is autism's environmental trigger."[40]

What about the age-old childhood disease of rickets, known to be caused by serious vitamin D deficiency?

"If adequate amounts of vitamin D prevent autism," speculates Cannell, "one would expect children with rickets to have an increased risk of autism."

While modern science has not yet run that comparison, Cannell found two old scientific papers predating 1943, when autism was first recognised and defined, that describe autism-like symptoms in children with rickets:

"Both papers describe 'weak mindedness', 'feeble minds', 'mental dullness', unresponsiveness and developmental delays. Even more intriguing, both papers report that the mental condition in rickets improved with vitamin D."[41]

39   "Vitamin D and autism: Clinical review," Kocovská et al, *Research in Developmental Disabilities*, Volume 33, Issue 5, September–October 2012, Pages 1541–1550

40   "Autism Spectrum Disorders Following In Utero Exposure To Antiepileptic Drugs," M. L. Evatt, *Neurology*, September 22, 2009 vol. 73 no. 12 997

41   "On the aetiology of autism," John Cannell, *Acta Paediatrica*

In 2010, Cannell threw down the gauntlet to health authorities: "Prove me wrong." To date, no conflicting evidence has emerged.

"Vitamin D induces more than 3,000 genes, many of which have a role in fetal development,[42]" wrote two Harvard University doctors to the *New England Journal of Medicine*.[43] "Vitamin D may be particularly relevant to the 'developmental origins hypothesis' described by Barker et al, in which environmental factors such as vitamin D may influence the genomic programming of fetal development and hence subsequent disease risk in both childhood and adult life."

In 1989, the American Medical Association issued an advisory to mothers about the high risk of letting sunlight fall on their children: "Keep infants out of the sun as much as possible". The years that followed have seen a huge increase in children diagnosed with autistic spectrum disorder and attention deficit hyperactivity disorder. Behavioural problems have soared. Could it all be linked?

"If this theory is true," Cannell said, "the path towards effective prevention – and perhaps [even] a treatment

2010; 99, Issue 8:1128-1130, http://onlinelibrary.wiley.com/doi/10.1111/j.1651-2227.2010.01883.x/full

42   "Transcriptomic analysis of human lung development," Kho et al, *American Journal of Respiratory Critical Care Medicine*, 2010; 181:54-63

43   "Letters, Vitamin D Insufficiency." Weiss S & Litonjua A, *NEJM* 364:14, April 7 2011, page 1379

effect if adequate physiological doses of vitamin D are given – is so simple, so safe, so inexpensive, so readily available and so easy, that it defies imagination.

"Seventeen vitamin D experts recently stated, 'In our opinion, children with chronic illnesses such as autism, diabetes and/or frequent infections should be supplemented with higher doses of sunshine or vitamin D3, doses adequate to maintain their 25(OH)D levels in the mid-normal of the reference range (65 ng/ml or 162 nmol/L) – and should be so supplemented year round'.

"Finally, if true, a darker side of the theory emerges. To some real but unknown extent, autism is an iatrogenic disease, caused by governments, organisations, committees, newspapers and physicians who promulgated the current warnings about sun exposure for pregnant women and young children without any understanding of the tragedy they engendered."

If true, the sun-safe slip, slop, slap campaign will go down as the deadliest and costliest public health mistake in history, having consigned millions to a needless life of autism and disability or, as we are about to discover, even worse.

Chapter 4

ASTHMA & ALLERGIES

"One in five of the babies was born with levels of less than 25 nmol/L (10 ng/ml), thus being seriously deficient"

– Study of NZ births by Dr Carlos Camargo,
Massachusetts General Hospital, 2011

Most of us know someone who has suffered with asthma or allergies. Some of us, as parents, have watched our children puff and wheeze and drain the life-giving drugs out of asthma inhalers. Roughly one in eight people reading this will directly suffer from asthma at some point in their lives.[44] Around one in every 200 of you will die from it.[45]

There have been a number of causes cited for asthma,

---

44   Centers for Disease Control and Prevention. National Center for Health Statistics. National Health Interview Survey Raw Data, 1997-2009.

45   "The Burden of Asthma in New Zealand", Holt S & Beasley R, Asthma & Respiratory Foundation of NZ, December 2001

from diet, vaccinations and even recent studies warning that paracetamol could trigger asthma attacks in children. As you might have gathered from the book so far, there's a distinct possibility that the published list of possible causes are what we might call 'final causes', the straw that broke the camel's back on the day. The reason the camel was vulnerable, however, may well have been a failure to sunbathe.

Just as there's strong evidence that vitamin D in fetal development is crucial for lowering the risk of autistic spectrum disorders, it seems equally likely that vitamin D plays the same role in preparing fetal immune systems and organ development.

We've seen that unlike most vitamins, vitamin D (which is actually a secosteroid, not a real vitamin) has built in reception areas throughout the human body, known as vitamin D receptors or VDRs. Additionally, those docking bays and pathways have now been mapped to more than 3,000 genes in the human body, with new VDRs being discovered all the time. The human body, it transpires, craves vitamin D so it makes sense those 3,000 genes might start playing up if they don't get their fix.

It's hard to imagine that fifteen years ago scientists knew virtually nothing of this. All over the world, while your eyes are scanning this sentence, somewhere on the globe research teams are beavering away, effectively in 24/7 mode, trying to unlock just how significant vitamin D might be for human health.

In the case of asthma, very.

It's the nation of New Zealand that's been at the cutting edge of some of this work. Back in the 1960s, New Zealand suffered an explosion of asthma deaths, and again in the 1980s. As an agricultural producer whose food and wines are consumed all over the world, the country pioneered high technology farming and production techniques. Of necessity, advances were sometimes hit and miss until the right formulations were found. One of those areas of experimentation was herbicides and pesticides.

The giant US company Dow Chemicals was a big supplier to New Zealand, and in fact helped manufacture the two key components of the Vietnam War defoliant known as "Agent Orange" from its factory at New Plymouth, on New Zealand's west coast. A former director of that company told *Investigate* magazine in 2000 that his company had not only shipped 2,4,5-T and 2,4-D off to be mixed into Agent Orange for the Vietnam War, but they'd also marketed the same mix to New Zealand farmers as a tough farm herbicide.[46]

The magazine found numerous instances of birth defects in farming children, and it's not hard to imagine that one of the nastiest chemicals in the sixties found its way onto the dinnerplates of all New Zealand

46   *Investigate* magazine, Jan/Feb 2001, pp26-33, http://www. investigatemagazine.com/pdf%27s/jan2.pdf

children at the time simply by being dropped on farms and then working its way up the food chain. Thus, a previous boom in asthma mortality coincident with this dark period is not entirely surprising.

Additionally, with vast pine plantations and farmland creating plenty of pollen, New Zealand had perfectly natural reasons for rising asthma rates.

Leaving aside those spikes, what those asthma epidemics triggered, however, was ground breaking research into the origins of the disease. Once again, it appears that vitamin D lays the groundwork for whether you or your children are biologically fortified against irritants.

The world, as we know, is full of irritants, but scientists are gradually coming to realise that the irritants are only taking advantage of existing weaknesses that shouldn't be there.

All of us are exposed, but not all of us develop asthma, eczema or allergies. Just as some people can happily smoke every day and live to a hundred, many more of us are genetically programmed to cark it if we take up smoking. The whole point of public health campaigns is that they address the needs of the majority, or significant minority. They cannot account for occasional exceptions.

In asthma's case, environmental factors appear to target a certain percentage of individuals. The final trigger may be ill-defined or different in various sufferers, but the result is the same. Maybe there's something that can predict your risk of developing asthma, however.

In 2010, Harvard University Professor of Medicine Dr Carlos Camargo Jr led a research team focusing on a promising new data sample: umbilical cord blood from 922 newborn babies in New Zealand. With the second highest rate of asthma in the world, behind the UK, Camargo and team wanted to test a promising new hypothesis, that maternal intake of vitamin D during pregnancy reduced the risk of wheezing and asthma in children. Cord blood, they figured, would provide definitive proof at the moment of birth of actual vitamin D levels.

The average vitamin D level in the blood was only 44 nmol/L, or less than 20 ng/ml. In other words, across 922 babies born in the cities of Wellington and Christchurch, New Zealand, at latitudes 41S and 43S respectively,[47] the average vitamin D level was in the "deficient" zone. One in five of the babies was born with levels of less than 25 nmol/L (10 ng/ml), thus being "seriously deficient".

What did they find?

Babies born with seriously deficient vitamin D levels were nearly 2.4 times more likely to have suffered an infection before the age of three months, in comparison with babies in the highest group who had levels in excess of 75 nmol/L (30 ng/ml, the minimum adequate

---

47   As a reference point, Boston is at latitude 42N.

range). The most deficient babies were more than twice as likely to have suffered a respiratory infection before the age of three months.[48]

The research team speculated that newborns with low vitamin D may be more susceptible to infections of any kind, because vitamin D is known to stimulate the production of natural antibiotics within the human body, and in particular cathelicidin, an "antimicrobial peptide" that is produced to protect bronchial passages as part of the immune defence system.[49]

By definition, low vitamin D = low immunity.

"Interventions to improve vitamin D status [in pregnancy] may provide a simple, safe and inexpensive way to reduce the respiratory infections that cause most asthma exacerbations," reported the researchers.

Recent studies, they wrote, have shown that asthmatic children with higher levels of vitamin D suffer fewer serious asthma attacks. A Japanese study, for example, found vitamin D supplements of 1200IU a day given to school students with a history of asthma resulted in an

---

48   "Cord blood 25-hydroxyvitamin D levels and risk of respiratory infection, wheezing and asthma," Camargo et al, *Pediatrics* 2011, Vol 127, Issue 1:e180-e187

49   "Induction of cathelicidin in normal and CF bronchial epithelial cells by 1,25-dihydroxyvitamin D(3)", Yim et al, *Journal of Cystic Fibrosis*, 2007; 6(6):403-410. See also "UVB radiation induces the expression of antimicrobial peptides in human keratinocytes in vitro and in vivo," Glaser et al, *Journal of Allergy & Clinical Immunology* 2009; 123(5):1117-1123

83% reduction in their risks of catching Influenza A.[50]

The low vitamin D status of New Zealand newborns also turned out to be an indicator of wheezing outbreaks by the age of 5. Children with the lowest vitamin D had more than double the risk of developing wheezing by their fifth birthday.

Announcing their findings, Camargo and team reported that one in five "apparently healthy" New Zealand children started life with vitamin D levels below 10 ng/ml. "These low levels were associated with a higher risk of respiratory infection during the first months of life and a higher risk of cumulative wheeze throughout early childhood."

The team couldn't find any specific link to full blown asthma by age five, but a unit across the Tasman Sea in Australia did.

In 2011, researchers from the University of Western Australia made a breakthrough discovery in a study of nearly 2,400 asthma sufferers under the age of 15. Blood serum levels of vitamin D were checked in 989 six year olds and 1,380 14-year-olds.[51]

---

50   "Randomized trial of vitamin D supplementation to prevent seasonal influenza A in schoolchildren", Urashima et al, *American Journal of Clinical Nutrition*, March 10, 2010 doi: 10.3945/ ajcn.2009.29094, http://www.anaboliclabs.com/User/Document/ Articles/Vitamin%20D/11.%20Urashima,%20Vit%20D,%202010.pdf
51   "Vitamin D and atopy and asthma phenotypes in children: a longitudinal cohort study", Hollams et al, *European Respiratory Journal*, December 2011, Vol 38 No. 6:1320-1327

After running the data for analysis, they found that low vitamin D levels at the age of six were a "significant predictor" of allergy sensitivity and developing asthma by the age of 14.

"Children, particularly males, with inadequate vitamin D are at increased risk of developing atopy [allergic sensitivity], and subsequently bronchial hyper-responsiveness and asthma."

Analysing these results from Australasia, Dr Scott Weiss of Harvard University's Channing Laboratory wrote that the Hollams study out of Australia was the first in the world to demonstrate an association between vitamin D levels at age 6 and asthma by age 14, and was one of "the first using [actual] vitamin D levels as a biomarker of vitamin D exposure".[52]

Weiss said the New Zealand study by Camargo et al filled in the blanks of the first five years of life, which the Hollams study didn't cover.

The evidence on asthma, he noted, was strong enough to justify full clinical trials of vitamin D as part of the inhalant mix for asthmatics, and those trials are now underway. But he warned that whilst higher vitamin D during pregnancy appears to reduce the incidence of asthma, it does not eliminate it completely, and should the trials clarify the issue, "some degree of post-natal

---

52 "Vitamin D in asthma and allergy: what next?", Weiss S & Litonjua A, *European Respiratory Journal*, December 2011, Vol 38 No. 6:1255-1257

supplementation will also probably be necessary to maintain normal immune function in the long term."

In 2012, the Arab emirate of Qatar corroborated the Australasian studies, noting vitamin D deficiency is "the major predictor of Asthma in Qatari children".[53] Researchers found those with the lowest levels were 482% – almost five times – more likely to suffer asthma. Coming from a family with low vitamin D levels was also a risk factor for asthmatic children – possible evidence of the dangers when sun avoidance practices become intergenerational.

In July 2012, a study of 1024 asthmatic American children in a random trial found those with high vitamin D levels had twice as much health benefit from their corticosteroid asthma medication as children with low vitamin D, illustrating that the vitamin enhanced the effect of the medicine.[54]

Asthma, allergies and respiratory problems are not the only things that vitamin D may protect you from in the chest area.

53   "Vitamin D deficiency as a strong predictor of asthma in children," Bener et al, *International Archives of Allergy and Immunology*, 2012; 157(2):168-175

54   "The Effect of Vitamin D and Inhaled Corticosteroid Treatment on Lung Function in Children", Wu et al, *Am. J. Respir. Crit. Care Med.* July 12, 2012 rccm.201202-0351OC

Chapter 5

CANCER, BREAST

"High vitamin D levels at early breast cancer diagnosis correlate with lower tumour size and better overall survival"
– findings published in Carcinogenesis, 2012

Each year, more than 200,000 women in the USA, 14,000 from Australia, 22,000 Canadians, 48,000 Brits and 2,500 in New Zealand are diagnosed with breast cancer. Roughly one in five victims die from it or related complications over time – the most recent figures from 2008 disclose a global death toll of 458,000 people that year. In the western world, around one in every eight women will develop breast cancer during their lifetime.

For all of the above reasons, and the huge financial cost, and community and personal trauma associated with cancer, there are very good reasons for seizing hold of anything that could reduce the incidence of breast cancer or improve survival rates from it.

If you do a search in Google Scholar for the phrases breast cancer and vitamin D, it'll throw up more than 58,000 references. Studies are pouring out literally every week, not just because the research on vitamin D has been so promising, but also because the early studies were flawed.

Here's an example. In 2008, researchers disclosed how they'd given 36,000 American women either a daily supplement of vitamin D and calcium, or a placebo, as part of research into bone fractures carried out by the Women's Health Initiatives. The icing on the cake was the sample was also large enough to catch subsets of women who subsequently developed cancer over the seven year trial period.

The study – one of the largest randomised controlled trials – found no difference in invasive breast cancer between those on the vitamin D supplements and those on the placebo.[55] It also looked for a protective effect in women who developed colorectal cancer, and found no benefit there either.[56]

Federal health agencies in various countries used this study to declare that "the science is not settled" on the benefits of vitamin D, but in truth they'd fallen victim

55 "Calcium Plus Vitamin D Supplementation and the Risk of Breast Cancer," Chlebowski et al, *J Natl Cancer Inst* Volume 100, Issue 22:1581-1591
56 "Calcium plus vitamin D supplementation and the risk of colorectal cancer," Wactawski-Wende et al, *N Engl J Med*. 2006 Feb 16;354(7):684-96

to human error. The problem with the vitamin D study wasn't that the vitamin had no benefit, but that the supplements they'd given the women contained too little of the vitamin to make a difference against cancer, and/or, they had not properly adjusted for women who were already taking vitamin D before the trial started.

Those supplements in the trial contained only 400IU of vitamin D3, which scientists now admit was like throwing one bucket of water on a house fire. Additionally in a study measuring change there was unlikely to be any change if many of the women were already on supplements earlier.

In 2011, researchers re-adjusted for precisely that error and found that – despite the low 400IU dose – there was in fact a change:

"In 15,646 women (43%) who were not taking personal calcium or vitamin D supplements at randomization, [the Vitamin D plus Calcium dose] significantly decreased the risk of total, breast, and invasive breast cancers by 14–20% and nonsignificantly reduced the risk of colorectal cancer by 17%."[57]

As you'll see, the cancer risk reduction, despite being good, isn't a patch on what was achieved with higher doses of vitamin D3.

---

57   "Calcium and vitamin D supplements and health outcomes: a reanalysis of the Women's Health Initiative (WHI) limited-access data set," Bolland et al, *Am J Clin Nutr* October 2011 vol. 94 no. 4 1144-1149

To cover the totality of research would take an encyclopedia, rather than a book. Instead, let's examine simply some of the most recent studies.

In May 2012, the journal *Carcinogenesis* reported on a Belgian study that measured the blood serum vitamin D levels of nearly 1,800 women when they were initially diagnosed with breast cancer, and then compared the course of the disease with their initial vitamin D status.[58]

This wasn't a trial measuring supplements, but instead directly measuring the blood levels of vitamin D which, of course, is the ultimate point. You take supplements, or sunbathe, in order to raise your blood levels of vitamin D.

Women with the highest levels of vitamin D (above 30 ng/ml or 75 nmol/L) when first diagnosed, managed to cut by half their risk of dying within five years, when compared with women who had vitamin D levels below 30 ng/ml. Further nailing the link to vitamin D, every 10 ng/ml rise in levels on diagnosis gave that patient an average 20% reduction in risk of dying within five years.

The researchers found the massive drop in the mortality rate remained intact even after making allow-

---

58   "Vitamin D status at breast cancer diagnosis: correlation with tumor characteristics, disease outcome and genetic determinants of vitamin D insufficiency." Hatse et al, *Carcinogenesis*. 2012 May 24. [Epub ahead of print]

ances for other factors like body size that could have influenced survival rates.

Another big finding from the study was that women with the highest vitamin D levels had the smallest – and therefore most curable – tumours. That's important, because it showed high vitamin D levels appear to hamper tumour growth and slow down the spread of cancer cells.

Women with the highest levels also enjoyed the longest periods of remission, although this particular benefit only applied to post-menopausal women. Given that 60% of breast cancers strike after menopause, that's highly relevant. Researchers suspect the bodies of post-menopausal women use vitamin D in different ways as a result of lower estrogen. Unfortunately, women are far more likely to be deficient in vitamin D after menopause, making supplementation or sunlight all the more important in the fight against breast cancer.

In their conclusion, the *Carcinogenesis* researchers state: "High vitamin D levels at early breast cancer diagnosis correlate with lower tumor size and better OS [overall survival], and improve breast cancer-specific outcome, especially in postmenopausal patients."[59]

It's certainly not the first study to find women have

---

59   "Vitamin D status at breast cancer diagnosis," Hatse et al, *Carcinogenesis* 2012, published online 23 May, doi: 10.1093/carcin/bgs187

much better odds of beating cancer if they keep their vitamin D levels up. Joan Lappe's groundbreaking report in the *Journal of Clinical Nutrition* that followed more than 400 Nebraska women getting 1100IU of vitamin D daily for four years found they reduced their risk of cancer of any kind by 77% during that time, in comparison with the placebo group.[60]

A 2006 study tested the vitamin D levels of breast cancer sufferers against a control group and found women with less than 20 ng/ml (50 nmol/L) of vitamin D were three and a half times more likely to develop breast cancer.[61]

Precisely how vitamin D works against breast cancer is still being determined, but a 2010 study reports that when vitamin D was used against breast cancer cells in laboratory experiments, half the cells shrivelled up and died.

"What happens is that Vitamin D enters the cells and triggers the cell death process," researcher JoEllen Welsh told *Good Morning America*. "It's similar to

---

60   It's also a direct example of how different studies can be. The 2008 Women's Health Initiative study found 400IU daily of vitamin D made no difference, while nearly three times that dose in the 2007 study clearly did. See "Vitamin D and calcium supplementation reduces cancer risk," Lappe et al, *American Journal of Clinical Nutrition*, 2007, 85(6):1586-91, http://img2. tapuz.co.il/forums/1_153137280.pdf

61   "Vitamin D status and breast cancer risk," Colston et al, *Anticancer Res.* 2006 Jul-Aug;26(4A):2573-80

what we see when we treat cells with Tamoxifen."[62]

Vitamin D status may also determine how vulnerable you are to the nastier breast cancers. There are different types of tumour, and surgeons have to treat them differently. Roughly 75% are known as ER positive, meaning they grow bigger in response to estrogen. Treatment options like Tamoxifen work by helping to block the estrogen receptors (docking bays) that the breast cancer cells feed from.

If your cancer is ER negative, your treatment is more difficult and your prognosis is not as good.

A University of Rochester study has found breast cancer patients with "sub-optimal" vitamin D levels of less than 33 ng/ml in their blood, were more than two and a half times more likely to have a "more aggressive", ER negative tumour. Worse, if there could be such a thing, they were more than three times more likely to develop what's known as a "triple negative cancer", such tumours being unresponsive to drugs like Tamoxifen or Herceptin.[63]

"These cancers generally respond well to adjuvant chemotherapy. Overall, however, they have a poorer prognosis than other types of breast cancer. So far, no

62   "In tests, vitamin D shrinks breast cancer cells," by Suzan Clarke, *ABC News*, 22 Feb 2010

63   "The association between breast cancer prognostic indicators and serum 25-OH vitamin D levels," Peppone et al, *Annals of Surgical Oncology* 2012, doi: 10.1245/s10434-012-2297-3

targeted therapies like Tamoxifen or Herceptin have been developed to help prevent recurrence in women with triple-negative breast cancer. Cancer experts are studying several promising targeted strategies aimed at triple-negative breast cancer."[64]

The discovery that vitamin D is manufactured locally in breast cells is a vital clue, because it proves vitamin D is supposed to be found in breasts. There would be no biological reason for vitamin D production in healthy breast cells unless it served a purpose. This discovery makes the protective "effect of vitamin D in breast cancer biologically plausible."[65]

An intriguing new twist that further establishes vitamin D as central to fighting cancer has emerged from a study of black American women. It has long been known that people with darker skins have a harder time generating vitamin D in the cooler temperate zones, so if vitamin D is involved in cancer you'd expect darker skinned people to be hit harder.

Just as with autism, so with cancer. Not only are African-American women six times more likely to be vitamin D deficient, but they are also more likely to suffer from a faulty gene that interferes with vitamin D production. That leaves them particularly vulnerable

---

64   http://www.webmd.com/breast-cancer/breast-cancer-types-er-positive-her2-positive

65   "Vitamin D and breast cancer," Shao et al, *The Oncologist*, January 2012; Vol 17(1):36-45

to the more aggressive "ER negative" form of breast cancer, which again fits with the study mentioned a moment ago.

Those African-American women who beat the odds and had the highest levels of vitamin D turn out to have a further variation that actually cut their aggressive breast cancer risk by half.

What does this mean? It shows that the rates of the most untreatable breast cancers in dark-skinned women appear to be linked to genetic variations in how they are able to process vitamin D. Once again, this humble, long-forgotten vitamin is at the centre of a revolution in how we understand the rise of cancer in modern times.

Scientists are now beginning to wonder what happens if teenage girls don't get enough sun or vitamin D while their breasts are developing. Researchers have gone back to a group of 29,480 women interviewed as teenagers way back in 1998 as part of the Nurses' Health Study.

Of that sample, 682 have since developed what's known as proliferative benign breast disease. Women with the highest dietary intakes of vitamin D foods in 1998 turn out to have reduced their risk of benign breast disease by 21%, leading the study to conclude, "vitamin D intake during adolescence may be important in the earlier stage of breast carcinogenesis [and offer] new pathways and strategies for breast cancer prevention."[66]

66   "Adolescent intakes of vitamin D and calcium and incidence of

Another recent study looked at the differences between pre-menopausal and post-menopausal breast cancer sufferers. Again, they found undeniable evidence that lower vitamin D equals a worse outcome. The study covered 2,000 women aged 35 to 69, half diagnosed with breast cancer and half of them in the control group.

Women with 30 ng/ml (75 nmol/L) of vitamin D were found to have only half the risk of developing breast cancer as women with 20 ng/ml (50 nmol/L) – currently regarded as an "adequate" level of vitamin D by health authorities in some countries like New Zealand.

When they looked at the split, pre- and post menopause, they found younger women with good vitamin D cut their risk of developing breast cancer by 40%, while older women enjoyed a 63% risk reduction.[67]

Those are huge numbers in the great scheme of things. And in the great scheme of things, they do actually mean something. It's true that full randomised, double-blind trials on people to see whether they develop cancer or not are pretty rare. The Women's Health Initiative RCT was too low-dose to really shine. What's needed is a study using doses of 4000IU or 5000IU a

proliferative benign breast disease", Su et al, *Breast Cancer Research & Treatment* 2012, doi: 10.1007/s10549-012-2091-8

67   "Serum 25-hydroxyvitamin D and risk of breast cancer: results of a large population-based case-control study in Mexican women," Fedirko et al, *Cancer Causes And Control*, 2012, Vol 23(7):1149-1162

day. But there have been many studies showing women with high vitamin D levels have a much greater chance of surviving breast cancer, or not developing it at all.

"Prevention of breast cancer is one of the greatest challenges currently facing public health researchers and policymakers," reported an analysis in 2011.[68]

"Globally, a wide range of epidemiologic studies have shown an inverse relationship between sunlight or UV B (UVB) irradiance (the main source of circulating vitamin D in humans),1-8 oral vitamin D intake,9-14 and serum 25-hydroxyvitamin D [25(OH) D] concentration (the main circulating vitamin D metabolite),15-22 with risk of breast cancer.

"There is also substantial laboratory evidence that vitamin D metabolites exert several powerful anti-carcinogenic effects on breast cancer cells."

The analysts, in their study funded by the US Navy, also make the point that public health agencies have acted in the past on the basis of evidence staring them in the face, without waiting for randomized trials in every case:

"Epidemiological history has shown that an RCT is not necessary to establish causality or to prevent a disease. For example, it is widely accepted that tobacco

---

68   "Does the evidence for an inverse relationship between serum vitamin D status and breast cancer risk satisfy the Hill criteria?", Mohr et al, *Dermato-Endocrinology*, Volume 4, Issue 2, April/ May/June 2012, http://www.es.landesbioscience.com/journals/ dermatoendocrinology/2012DE0186.pdf

smoking causes lung cancer, yet this knowledge was gained as the result of ordinary observational studies."

Observational studies also found the cause of cholera, and helped in contact tracing for tuberculosis.

"Furthermore, RCT's take far longer to complete and can cost up to 350 times as much as a nested case-control or ordinary case control study of the same topic when the purpose is testing prevention.

"Study after study, utilizing varying designs in both human populations and the laboratory, has demonstrated that vitamin D substantially reduces the risk of breast cancer. The A.B. Hill criteria have been largely satisfied, providing a compelling case for a causal, inverse relationship between vitamin D status and risk of breast cancer."

Those arguments are backed up by the conclusions of a 2011 study into the most aggressive breast cancers, which found a 63% reduction in risk for breast cancer overall:

"In our analyses, higher serum levels of 25OHD were associated with reduced risk of breast cancer, with associations strongest for high grade, ER negative or triple negative cancers in premenopausal women. With further confirmation in large prospective studies, these findings could warrant vitamin D supplementation for reducing breast cancer risk, particularly those with poor prognostic characteristics among premenopausal women.[69]

---

69   "Pretreatment Serum Concentrations of 25-Hydroxyvitamin

"Because the risk of triple negative breast cancer peaks before menopause, and because vitamin D deficiency can be easily corrected by increasing sun exposure and/or supplement intake, if our findings are confirmed in large prospective studies for temporal causality, vitamin D may be used as a potential cancer preventive agent against triple negative cancers among young women."

Note that they feel the results are getting strong enough to warrant using vitamin D as a cautionary preventative, much as low dose aspirin has been used for cardiovascular disease.

Another team looking at this issue admits there is a difference in opinion between health policy officials, and specialists working at the coal face:[70]

"25-OH vitamin D is the accepted assessment of vitamin D status and provides a comprehensive measure of vitamin D from all sources (diet, sunlight, and supplementation). Although there is not a 'standard' definition of vitamin D status, a widely accepted classification is deficiency at <20 ng/ml, insufficiency at

D and Breast Cancer Prognostic Characteristics: A Case-Control and a Case-Series Study," Yao et al, *PLoS ONE* 6(2): e17251. doi:10.1371/journal.pone.0017251, http://www.plosone.org/article/info%3Adoi%2F10.1371%2Fjournal.pone.0017251

70   "The effect of various vitamin D supplementation regimens in breast cancer patients", Peppone et al, *Breast Cancer Research & Treatment*, Volume 127, Number 1 (2011), 171-177, http://www.ncbi.nlm.nih.gov/pmc/articles/PMC3085185/

20–31 ng/ml, and an optimal range of ≥32 ng/ml.[71] "Despite a number of clinical trials, researchers and clinicians remain divided on the proper supplementation amount to achieve a normal 25-OH vitamin D level. The current recommendation by the Food and Nutrition Board (FNB) of the Institute of Medicine is for 400 IU a day of vitamin D for adults, with 2,000 IU a day as the tolerable upper intake level.

"However, numerous clinical trials administering low-dose vitamin D supplementation (≤800 IU/day) to participants with sub-optimal vitamin D levels failed to achieve optimal 25-OH vitamin D levels.[72] A recent study of breast cancer patients receiving treatment found supplementation with almost 2,000 IU a day of vitamin D failed to normalize 25-OH levels in

71 "Vitamin D insufficiency in North America," Hanley et al, *J Nutr.* 2005;135:332–337 See also: "Redefining vitamin D insufficiency," Malabanan et al, *Lancet.* 1998;351:805–806. See also: "Estimates of optimal vitamin D status", Dawson-Hughes et al, *Osteoporos Int.* 2005;16:713–716

72 "Vitamin D status and effect of low-dose cholecalciferol and high-dose ergocalciferol supplementation in multiple sclerosis," Hiremath et al. *Mult Scler.* 2009;15:735–740, See also "Vitamin D supplementation and fracture incidence in elderly persons. A randomized, placebo-controlled clinical trial," Lips et al, *Ann Intern Med.* 1996;124:400–406. See also "Can vitamin D supplementation reduce the risk of fracture in the elderly? A randomized controlled trial," Meyer et al, *J Bone Miner Res.* 2002;17:709–715. See also "High prevalence of vitamin D deficiency despite supplementation in premenopausal women with breast cancer undergoing adjuvant chemotherapy," Crew et al. *J Clin Oncol.* 2009;27:2151–2156

50% of participants.[73] Vitamin D deficient individuals often require a short course (4–16 weeks) of high-dose vitamin D supplementation (≥40,000 IU/week) to achieve an optimal 25-OH vitamin D level, although experimental evidence is severely limited.[74] While the FNB defines 2,000 IU a day of vitamin D as the upper intake level, high-dose vitamin D supplementation is well tolerated among a variety of participant popula-tions, including those with cancer."[75]

It seems pretty clear then that small doses of vitamin D are not enough to help cancer patients, and that some fairly serious prescribed supplements of up to 40,000IU a week may be necessary to compensate for initial vitamin D deficiency.

---

73   "Vitamin D threshold to prevent aromatase inhibitor-induced arthralgia: a prospective cohort study.Prieto-Alhambra D, Javaid MK, Servitja S, Arden NK, Martinez-Garcia M, Diez-Perez A, Albanell J, Tusquets I, Nogues X. *Breast Cancer Res Treat.* 2011;125:869–878

74   "Diagnosis and treatment of vitamin D deficiency," Cannell et al, *Expert Opin Pharmacother.* 2008;9:107–118

75   "A phase 2 trial exploring the effects of high-dose (10, 000 IU/day) vitamin D(3) in breast cancer patients with bone metastases," Amir et al, *Cancer* 2010;116:284–291. See also "High-dose oral vitamin D3 supplementation in the elderly," Bacon et al, *Osteoporos Int.* 2009;20:1407–1415. See also "A phase I/II dose-escalation trial of vitamin D3 and calcium in multiple sclerosis," Burton et al, *Neurology.* 2010;74:1852–1859. See also "No significant effect on bone mineral density by high doses of vitamin D3 given to overweight subjects for one year," Jorde et al, *Nutr J.* 2010;9:1

Chapter 6

CANCER, COLON & PROSTATE

"People diagnosed with colorectal cancer in the summer and autumn, when 25(OH)D concentrations are highest, had significantly better survival than those diagnosed in the winter"

– Dr Kimmie Ng, Harvard, 2011

COLORECTAL CANCER

Like breast cancer, the science on bowel cancer, as it is commonly known, is being written every day. There's a lot riding on it. In 2008, an estimated 1.23 million people developed colorectal cancer, and more than 600,000 died from it, making it a bigger and more efficient killer than breast cancer.

In 2007, a review of published medical studies (known as a 'meta analysis') found that estimated blood levels of vitamin D of 33 ng/ml (82.5 nmol/L) were associated with a 50% lower risk of colon cancer.[76]

76   "Optimal vitamin D status for colorectal cancer prevention: a quantitative meta analysis," Gorham et al, *American Journal of*

A 2008 study of bowel cancer patients found those with the highest vitamin D levels in their blood when they were first diagnosed with cancer cut their risk of dying by 48% – these were patients who already had the disease. Once again, the higher the vitamin D, the better chance you have of beating bowel cancer.[77]

The US National Cancer Institute's main information page on vitamin D acknowledges that studies are showing benefits:

"At least one epidemiologic study has reported an association between vitamin D and reduced mortality from colorectal cancer. Among the 16,818 participants in the Third National Health and Nutrition Examination Survey,[78] those with higher vitamin D blood levels (≥80 nmol/L or 32ng/ml) had a 72 percent lower risk of colorectal cancer death than those with lower vitamin D blood levels (< 50 nmol/L or 20 ng/ml)."

The National Cancer Institute points out that most bowel cancers begin with benign tumours known as adenomas, and that higher levels of vitamin D in the

Preventive Medicine 2007; 32(3):210-16

77   "Circulating 25-Hydroxyvitamin D Levels and Survival in Patients With Colorectal Cancer," Ng et al, *Journal of Clinical Oncology* June 20, 2008 vol. 26 no. 18 2984-2991. See also, "Prospective study of predictors of vitamin D status and survival in patients with colorectal cancer," Ng et al, *British Journal of Cancer*, 2009 Sep 15;101(6):916-23

78   "Prospective study of serum vitamin D and cancer mortality in the United States", Freedman et al, *Journal of the National Cancer Institute* 2007; 99(21):1594–1602

blood appear to lower the risk of adenomas developing. An NCI-sponsored study into the effect of diet on adenomas recurring after a colonoscopy was also able to monitor dietary intake for vitamin D – both through food and through supplements. The NCI reports the study found vitamin D gained solely from food appeared too trivial to have a beneficial effect, but that "individuals who used any amount of vitamin D supplements had a lower risk of adenoma recurrence."[79]

"In another study, the vitamin D intakes of 3,000 people from several Veterans Affairs medical centers were examined to determine whether there was an association between intake and advanced colorectal neoplasia (an outcome that included high-risk adenomas as well as colon cancer). Individuals with the highest vitamin D intakes (more than 16 µg, or 645 IU, per day) had a lower risk of developing advanced neoplasia than those with lower intakes.[80]

"A pooled analysis of data from these and a number of other observational studies found that higher circulating levels of vitamin D and higher vitamin D intakes were associated with lower risks of colorectal adenoma."[81]

---

79   "The association of calcium and vitamin D with risk of colorectal adenomas," Hartman et al, *Journal of Nutrition* 2005; 135(2):252–259

80   "Risk factors for advanced colonic neoplasia and hyperplastic polyps in asymptomatic individuals," Lieberman et al, *Journal of the American Medical Association* 2003; 290(22):2959–2967

81   "Vitamin D and prevention of colorectal adenoma: A

The National Cancer Institute also notes that circulating blood levels of vitamin D might actually need to be quite high for protective purposes: "Another large, NCI-sponsored randomized, placebo-controlled trial explored the effects of calcium supplementation and blood levels of vitamin D on adenoma recurrence. Calcium supplementation reduced the risk of adenoma recurrence only in individuals with vitamin D blood levels above 73 nmol/L. Among individuals with vitamin D levels at or below this level, calcium supplementation was not associated with a reduced risk."[82]

There are many other factors that help you avoid or survive cancers of course – diet being one of them – but the point here is that vitamin D is operating over and above that. Clearly, some people with high levels die regardless (otherwise the risk reduction would be 100%), but doubling your odds of survival with the Big C is not something to be sneezed at.

Given bowel cancer's high mortality rate, however, there is evidence that people can't be too complacent. Like breast cancer, if your vitamin D levels are not already high at the point of diagnosis, it may be too

meta-analysis," Wei et al, *Cancer Epidemiology, Biomarkers, and Prevention* 2008; 17(11):2958–2969

82   "Vitamin D, calcium supplementation, and colorectal adenomas: Results of a randomized trial," Grau et al, *Journal of the National Cancer Institute* 2003; 95(23):1765–1771

late for vitamin D to play much of a role in keeping you alive. Waiting until you get cancer, before reaching for the mega supplement, could be a deadly oversight.

A study published 2011, involving patients with Stage IV bowel cancer that had metastasised through the body, found two things. Firstly, that only 10% of their patient sample still had vitamin D levels high enough to be useful, and secondly, that the cancers had taken most of the victims beyond the point of no return.

The researchers led by Kimmie Ng provided a thoughtful analysis:[83]

"In the United States, colorectal cancer mortality follows a latitudinal gradient, with higher mortality rates seen in individuals who reside at higher latitudes. A large observational study in Norway found that people diagnosed with colorectal cancer in the summer and autumn, when 25(OH)D concentrations are highest, had significantly better survival than those diagnosed in the winter.[84] We previously showed that higher prediagnosis plasma levels of 25(OH)D and higher

---

83   "Vitamin D Status in Patients With Stage IV Colorectal Cancer: Findings From Intergroup Trial N9741," Ng et al, *Journal of Clinical Oncology*, April 20, 2011 vol. 29 no. 12 1599-1606
84   "Solar radiation, vitamin D and survival rate of colon cancer in Norway," Moan et al, *Journal of Photochemistry & Photobiology*, 2005 Mar 1;78(3):189-93. See also "Vitamin D3 from sunlight may improve the prognosis of breast-, colon- and prostate cancer (Norway)," Robsahm et al, *Cancer Causes Control*. 2004 Mar;15(2):149-58

postdiagnostic 25(OH)D scores are associated with significant reductions in mortality among patients with established colorectal cancer, although, in those studies, a substantially greater proportion of the population had plasma 25(OH)D levels higher than 33 ng/mL.

"In this study, we did not detect an association between higher plasma 25(OH)D and patient outcome. It is possible that vitamin D may have limited impact on the natural history of colorectal cancer once it has metastasized. Preclinical data indicate that VDR expression is decreased in late stages of neoplasia,[85] perhaps leading to loss of response of colon tumor cells to vitamin D. Yet another potential explanation for the discrepant results is that our study had limited statistical power, with only a small number of patients with plasma 25(OH)D levels sufficient for a protective effect on cancer outcome."

Other studies, likewise, have found that high vitamin D levels of 30 ng/ml (75 nmol/L) or more going into a cancer episode play an important role in survival:

"The majority of epidemiologic studies consistently support an approximately 20–30% reduction in risk of colorectal cancer and adenomas comparing high to low intake categories of both calcium and vitamin D, although independent effects may not be adequately

---

85   "1,25-Dihydroxyvitamin D3 Receptor as a Marker of Human Colon Carcinoma Cell Line Differentiation and Growth Inhibition," Shabahang et al, *Cancer Res* August 15, 1993 53; 3712

separated. Less consistency exists on the dose–response relation for both nutrients. Intake of calcium of not more than 1000 mg/d and intake of vitamin D of 1000–2000 IU/d, achieving a level of at least 30 ng/mL, appear important for colorectal cancer prevention."[86]

CANCER, PROSTATE

Vitamin D's links to prostate cancer are mixed. Blood samples taken from 14,000 American doctors in what's known as the Physicians Health Study reveal those with vitamin D levels below 25 ng/ml (62.5 nmol/L) had more than double the risk of developing an aggressive, often lethal, form of prostate cancer.[87]

The researchers found some men had a genetic variation that made them even more susceptible – two and a half times more likely to be struck with aggressive prostate cancer – in combination with low vitamin D, but that if men with that same gene fault had high vitamin D they actually enjoyed a drop in their risk – not a rise – of between 60 and 70%.

Staggering stuff, that vitamin D could work that hard to out-muscle a gene fault.

---

86   "Calcium, vitamin D and colorectal cancer chemoprevention," Zhang and Giovannucci, *Best Practice & Research Clinical Gastroenterology*, Volume 25, Issue 4 , Pages 485-494, August 2011

87   "A prospective study of plasma vitamin D metabolites, vitamin D receptor polymorphisms, and prostate cancer," Li et al, *PLoS Med.* 2007 Mar;4(3):e103, http://www.ncbi.nlm.nih.gov/pmc/articles/PMC1831738/?tool=pubmed

What's more sobering is that 51% of male doctors were suffering vitamin D 'insufficiency' or 'deficiency' even during summer time (possibly a direct result of following the sun avoidance advice), rising to 77% who were insufficient or deficient during winter and spring. With those low levels, clearly more than half the men were at a much higher risk of aggressive prostate cancer.

"Our data suggest that a large proportion of the US men had suboptimal vitamin D status (especially during the winter/spring season), and both 25(OH)D and 1,25(OH)2D may play an important role in preventing prostate cancer progression," the study authors concluded.

Why do I say "mixed"? Because studies so far have not shown a link between vitamin D levels and the less-aggressive, more general and gentle prostate cancer. One recent report followed up the health outcomes of 1,260 men who'd been diagnosed with prostate cancer at some point after providing blood samples way back in 1993-1995. Of that sample, 114 men had "lethal outcomes" by March 2011.

Researchers found strong links between high vitamin D levels in the blood, and a 57% lower chance of contracting the most aggressive prostate cancers. However, they "found no statistically significant association" between vitamin D levels and "overall prostate cancer". From that, they concluded "vitamin D is relevant for lethal prostate cancer".[88]

---

88   "Vitamin D related genetic variation, plasma vitamin D, and

Adding to the "mixed" is a strange study from Finland, known as the Alpha Tocopherol, Beta Carotene (or ATBC) trial, where higher vitamin D levels in the blood were linked to an *increased* risk of aggressive prostate cancer.[89] The fly in the ointment with this study is that the sample were entirely men who actively smoked, aged from 50-69. That same sample was also used in a study showing an increased risk of pancreatic cancer.[90] So is the lesson we take from this supposed to be that smoking and vitamin D don't mix? Vitamin D expert William Grant suspects so.

"The best hypothesis for why Finnish smokers have higher incidence of pancreatic cancer with higher serum 25(OH)D levels is that the vitamin D-pancreatic cancer relation is different for smokers and nonsmokers."[91]

He makes the point that there may be other environmental factors muddying the trial, or even a genetic variation peculiar to Scandinavia, similar to the genetic

risk of lethal prostate cancer etc," Shui et al, *Journal of the National Cancer Institute*, 2012, 104(9):690-699

89   "Serum 25-Hydroxyvitamin D and Prostate Cancer Risk in a Large Nested Case-Control Study," Albanes et al, *Cancer Epidemiology, Biomarkers and Prevention*, July 22, 2011; doi: 10.1158/1055-9965.EPI-11-0403

90   "A prospective nested case-control study of vitamin D status and pancreatic cancer risk in male smokers," Stolzenberg-Solomon et al, *Cancer Research* 2006; 66(20):10213–10219

91   "Critique of the U-shaped serum 25-hydroxyvitamin D level-disease response relation," William Grant, *Dermato-Endocrinology* 1:6, 289-293; November/December 2009;

variations discovered in other races. There's also the problem that baseline vitamin D levels were very low in the Finnish men anyway, prompting this comment on one prostate cancer forum:

"These Scandinavian vitamin D studies drive me nuts. When half the men are deficient and most of the others have insufficiency, what is the definition of "High"?"[92]

The answer, possibly, Finnish men caught smoking vitamin D supplements.

In all seriousness, however, researchers do wonder whether starting with a really low vitamin D average has made a difference:

"As recently summarized by Li et al,[93] the Nordic study populations[94] were distinguished by the large proportion of men deficient for serum vitamin D (ie, with serum levels <50 nmol/L – approximately 50% of the men were deficient, compared with only 20% for the US study populations)."[95]

---

92   http://health.groups.yahoo.com/group/natural_prostate_treatments/message/22796

93   "A prospective study of plasma vitamin D metabolites, vitamin D receptor polymorphisms, and prostate cancer," Li et al *PLoS Med* . 2007 ; 4 (3): e103

94   "Prostate cancer risk and prediagnostic serum 25-hydroxyvitamin D levels (Finland)," Ahonen et al, *Cancer Causes Control* . 2000 ; 11 (9): 847 – 852. See also "Both high and low levels of blood vitamin D are associated with a higher prostate cancer risk: a longitudinal, nested case-control study in the Nordic countries," Tuohimaa et al, *Int J Cancer* 2004 ; 108 (1): 104 – 108

95   "Serum Vitamin D Concentration and Prostate Cancer Risk:

Another example of racial variations affecting vitamin D's impact on prostate cancer comes from a study by the US National Institutes of Health of African-American men, which found a genetic variation that may account for some of the disproportionate prostate cancer in that community.

One of the theories behind prostate cancer is that it is stimulated by a high calcium intake. Although most of the men they studied (82%) consumed less than the recommended daily intake of 1200 mg of calcium in the diet, nonetheless men with the highest calcium intake (>1059 mg/day) were more than twice as likely to develop prostate cancer as men with the lowest intake (<488 mg/day).

Vitamin D is, of course, a key regulator of calcium absorption.

African-Americans were found to carry a gene making them much more susceptible to calcium intake. The same gene is found in European and Hispanic populations to a lesser degree. Where it has appeared in European men, it has also shown an increased risk for prostate cancer in conjunction with higher vitamin D levels.[96]

A Nested Case – Control Study," Ahn, Albanes et al, *Journal of the National Cancer Institute*, 2008 Vol. 100, Issue 11 | June 4, 2008
96   "Polymorphisms in the vitamin D receptor gene, ultraviolet radiation, and susceptibility to
prostate cancer" Bodiwala et al, *Environ Mol Mutagen*. 2004. 43(2):121-127.

However, the US researchers say the amount of calcium involved exceeds what vitamin D would normally process in a day, so the risk pathway for calcium is likely to be another as yet undiscovered mechanism. They suspect this genetic anomaly may lie behind conflicting results in vitamin D/prostate studies.

"A positive effect of serum calcium on prostate cancer risk may confound the relationship between 25(OH)D and prostate cancer risk in some studies, which may account for some discrepant results in the literature."

One of those results was a 2008 study – also involving scientist Demetrius Albanes, that found a higher risk of aggressive prostate cancer among men with higher vitamin D levels, but it is noteworthy that the study authors did not consider calcium intake was relevant to the result: "Factors that were found not to confound the associations of interest included the following: ... vitamin D (<200, 200 – 399, 400 – 599, 600 – 799, 800 – 999, ≥ 1000 IU/d), and calcium (<750, 750 – 999, 1000 – 1499, 1500 – 1999, ≥ 2000 mg/d) intake."[97]

US cancer biologist Gary Schwartz has gone so far as to place in the scientific record his evidence indicating "that the recent association between prostate cancer and serum 25-OHD by Albanes et al. [the Finnish study] is

---

97   "Serum Vitamin D Concentration and Prostate Cancer Risk: A Nested Case – Control Study," Ahn, Albanes et al, *Journal of the National Cancer Institute*, 2008 Vol. 100, Issue 11 | June 4, 2008

due to confounding or interaction with serum calcium."[98] African-Americans who didn't have the gene variation and were not as susceptible to calcium had a reduced risk of prostate cancer, further strengthening the suspicion that the often-used Finnish data may be flawed because it's being skewed by genetics. Adding to the scientific confusion further, a study of Caucasian American men included those who had the genetic variant but found they were unaffected by it: "Conversely, in a U.S. study of non-Hispanic white men, we found no significant association between VDR Cdx2 genotype and advanced prostate cancer risk, regardless of sun exposure."[99]

Moral of the story? Talk to your doctor.

---

98   "Circulating Vitamin D and Risk of Prostate Cancer – Letter," Gary Schwartz, *Cancer Epidemiology, Biomarkers & Prevention*, January 2012 21; 247; doi: 10.1158/1055-9965.EPI-11-091

99   "Sun exposure, vitamin D receptor gene polymorphisms, and risk of advanced prostate cancer," John et al, *Cancer Res.* 2005. 65(12):5470-5479.

Chapter 7

THE HEART OF THE MATTER

"Researchers found those with the lowest vitamin D levels were three times more likely to die of heart disease, and two and a half times more likely to die of any cause"

– results of NHANES III study

Heart disease is the world's biggest natural killer. Each year it accounts for between one in three and one in four deaths. In the US, roughly one in every 300 people suffers a heart attack each year.[100] We've been invited to try the so-called Mediterranean diet rich in olive oil and red wine, but researchers are now beginning to suspect the real secret ingredient in the Mediterranean diet was actually sunlight.

In 2012, a major study of 'metabolic syndrome' heart patients in Europe which tracked their health for nearly eight years has found people with the highest levels of vitamin D reduced their risk of sudden death by a

100   http://www.cdc.gov/heartdisease/facts.htm

massive 85%. There's not a drug on the planet that can deliver those kinds of odds.[101]

Ninety-two percent of those taking part had what research teams called "sub-optimal" levels of vitamin D: below 75 nmol/L (30 ng/ml), and a total of 22% of the sample fell into the "severely deficient" category of less than 25 nmol/L (10 ng/ml).

Of the 1,801 patients being tracked, 462 died within the trial period. Those with the highest levels of vitamin D were 75% less likely to die of any cause (heart failure, road crash, meteorite strike, any cause of death at all) and 85% less likely to suffer a "sudden death". For people with 'optimal' vitamin D, there was a 76% reduction in the risk of dying from congestive heart disease during the 7.7 year follow-up period. The reduction in death rate followed a sliding scale depending on vitamin D levels.

Fifteen percent of all European adults are believed to have 'metabolic syndrome', which is linked with obesity, hypertension and faulty glucose and insulin metabolism. It is a known precursor to both type-2 diabetes and cardiovascular disease. Up to one in three Americans suffer from it. The significance of this 2012 heart mortality study is thus fairly obvious.

101   "Vitamin D levels predict all-cause and cardiovascular disease mortality in subjects with the metabolic syndrome: the Ludwigshafen Risk and Cardiovascular Health (LURIC) Study," Thomas et al, *Diabetes Care.* 2012 May;35(5):1158-64. Epub 2012 Mar 7.

Precisely how vitamin D works on the cardiovascular system is still under investigation – given that medical researchers have really only cottoned on to the vitamin's multiple benefits over the past fifteen years. However, one recent study shows a possible pathway. There's a chemical known as plasma renin which has been linked to higher mortality in heart disease.

Now, a Serbian study of 101 heart patients in a double blind trial of 2000IU vitamin D supplements daily has found a big impact of vitamin D on renin production. The results, presented to a cardiovascular conference this year, show that after six weeks, patients given the 2000IU of D daily saw their blood levels rise from an average of only 48 nmol/L (19.2 ng/ml) to 80 nmol/L (32 ng/ml). In contrast, the vitamin D levels of heart patients on the placebo dropped from 47 nmol/L average to 44 nmol/L (17.6 ng/ml) over the six week trial.

"Six weeks of [vitamin D] supplementation dropped plasma renin activity by 1.3 nmol/L per hour, while control patients saw a 2.4 nmol/L/hr rise over the same period," said study leader Rudolf de Boer.[102]

In terms of the big picture, harmful plasma renin levels dropped from 65 ng/L to 55 ng/L in vitamin D patients, while they rose from 56 to 72 ng/L in the placebo group.

Facing media questions about why this trial showed promise where the Women's Health Initiative study

---

102   "Vitamin D may help in HF," *MedPage Today*, 22 May 2012

showed no benefits from vitamin D, Zurich University's Dr Frank Ruschitzka told *MedPage Today* that
the US WHI study (referred to earlier in this book)
was "seriously underdosed" at 400IU a day, in comparison to 2000IU/day.

The *American Journal of Cardiology* has also recently
published a major study of 10,899 patients enrolled
in a University of Kansas cardiovascular programme
between 2004 and 2009. It found that people with
vitamin D above 30 ng/ml (75 nmol/L) reduced their
mortality risk by 61% compared with people whose
vitamin D levels were lower.[103]

In fact, people with low vitamin D were an incredible 164% more likely to die during the five year study
period.

"Vitamin D deficiency was associated with a significant risk of cardiovascular disease and reduced survival,"
wrote the study authors. "Vitamin D supplementation
was significantly associated with better survival."

The study did not just document vitamin D levels
on enrolment (baseline levels), it also kept a record of
where doctors decided to prescribe vitamin D as part
of treatment. In total, 29.7% of the sample had good

---

103   "Vitamin D deficiency and supplementation and relation
to cardiovascular health," Vacek et al, *American Journal of
Cardiology*, 2012; 109:359-363, http://www.trackyourplaque.com/
userdata/3038/file/Vitamin%20D%20and%20CVD%20-%20
AJC%20Feb%202012.pdf

vitamin D levels, and 70.3% (7,665 patients) had low vitamin D. Of the 10,899 patients, a sub group of 2,423 who were vitamin D deficient at baseline were given supplements by their doctors each week. Some were given 1000IU a day, and others 50,000IU every fortnight, but the overall average across the subgroup was 2,254IU/day. These "deficient" patients given vitamin D supplements reduced their overall mortality risk – they still were 46% more likely to die than patients whose vitamin D levels had been high right from the start, but compare that with the "deficient" patients who were not given vitamin D supplements: their mortality risk increased by a massive 272%!

Vitamin D deficient heart patients were nearly three times more likely to die, and more than two and a quarter times more likely to develop diabetes mellitus, than patients whose vitamin D levels had been high from day one. They were nearly one and a half times more likely to develop high blood pressure.

Whilst this trial was not random or double-blind, because doctors made the choice to intervene and include high dose vitamin D as part of their cardio-vascular treatment arsenal, it does clearly show three main sample groups: those who had high vitamin D to begin with; those who had deficient levels of vitamin D to begin with; and finally those who were deficient but whose doctors decided to treat with vitamin D, additional to their other heart medication.

Vitamin D expert Dr John Cannell once threw down a challenge to his medical colleagues:

"Should practitioners routinely screen and aggressively treat vitamin D deficiency in patients with serious or potentially fatal illnesses, or should such patients [be left to] combat their disease vitamin D deficient?"[104]

It looks like the University of Kansas answered that challenge, and in doing so proved his point.

In the final analysis, those with the highest vitamin D levels from day one had the best survival rates. Those who were deficient but later given supplements had the biggest improvement in their survival rates. Those who relied on traditional heart drugs without treating their vitamin D deficiency were overwhelmingly the most likely to die within five years.

The study sends another clear signal that getting the public's vitamin D levels up is crucial, if people are to have the best chance of surviving major health scares. As you have seen so far in this book, people whose vitamin D levels are good *before* they are diagnosed with major disease are the real winners.

"Because vitamin D deficiency is widespread," note the study authors, "strategies directed at population-based supplementation programmes could prove beneficial."

Like the European team before them, the American researchers put previous "inconclusive" study results

---

104   http://0101.nccdn.net/1_5/3a0/1e8/00e/Cannell-Vitamin-D-study.pdf

down to bad design of the studies: "It is possible that the lack of benefit in these studies resulted from sub-optimal levels of vitamin D supplementation...400 to 800IU...which might not be adequate to ensure optimal serum levels."

A more "appropriate" daily dose for the public is "1000 to 2000IU", they suggest.

"Our findings are consistent with [previous] studies, suggesting poorer patient outcomes for patients with vitamin D deficiency. In addition, our data further extended these findings by demonstrating better sur-vival with vitamin D supplementation.

"The benefits of vitamin D supplementation on sur-vival were significant for those patients with a docu-mented deficiency. This benefit was independent of the concomitant use of other cardioprotective drugs such as aspirin or statins."

The comment about statins raises another important finding. Another study has found statins play a huge role in boosting the power of vitamin D in the body, leading one researcher[105] to suggest there is a possibil-ity "that some – or all – of the mortality reduction of statins may be mediated through increases in vitamin D levels."

Did heart patients with high vitamin D survive longer

---

105   "Use of vitamin D in clinical practice," Cannell & Hollis, *Alternative Medicine Review*, March 2008, Vol 13(1), http://0101. nccdn.net/1_5/3a0/1e8/00e/Cannell-Vitamin-D-study.pdf

because the vitamin made the statins more effective?

A stunning new twist in this emerged in 2009. A group of Turkish researchers studying the effects of statins at a hospital in Ankara were stunned at an unexpected side-effect of their study. A group of mostly Muslim women were taking part in an eight week trial of rosuvastatin therapy. When their blood was tested, the 25(OH)D levels had risen from an average of 14 ng/ml to 36.3 ng/ml over the eight weeks. These people were not on vitamin D supplements, it was winter, and most of them wore full garb. The kind of vitamin D increase they enjoyed is not normally seen without massive vitamin D supplementation or lots of summer sun.

Staggered, the researchers organised a second, randomized controlled trial of a similar population sample at the same hospital, in the same months of a different year. They threw in a different statin, fluvastatin, in order to see whether the effect was common or specific to the rosuvastatin.

At the end of eight weeks, the rosuvastatin group had, again, increased their blood serum vitamin D from 11.8 ng/ml to 35.2 ng/ml. There was no significant rise in the fluvastatin group.

"We propose that some statins may be increasing the absorption of vitamin D by stimulating the expressions of cholesterol transporters," wrote the study authors in 2012. "This effect, which was shown with atorvastatin, can be studied with rosuvastatin, and may open up a horizon to explain the link between statins and vitamin D."[106]

From that study, it certainly appears that some statins are using vitamin D to weave magic in the body.

One way that vitamin D doesn't appear to affect the heart is through influence on the arteries. A University of Wisconsin team speculated that the vitamin reduced arterial "stiffness", and gave 114 women a cookie each day. Half the sample had biscuits laced with 2500IU of vitamin D, and the other half just ordinary biscuits. After four months, they found no impact on arterial stiffness or blood pressure.[107]

That's not always the way the cookie crumbles, however. A Danish study of 112 patients – half given 3000IU of vitamin D and half a placebo – found that over 20 weeks in winter, systolic and diastolic blood pressure measurements lowered significantly, by 7 and 2 points respectively.[108]

To put that in perspective for the ordinary reader, the

106   "Statins and vitamin D: a hot topic that will be discussed for a long time," Yavuz & Ertugrul, *Dermato-Endocrinology*, Vol 4, Issue 1, Jan/Feb/Mar 2012

107   "A Prospective Randomized Controlled Trial of the Effects of Vitamin D Supplementation on Cardiovascular Disease Risk," Gepner et al, *PLoS One*, 7(5): e36617. doi:10.1371/journal. pone.0036617

108   "Vitamin D Supplementation During Winter Months Reduces Central Blood Pressure In Patients With Hypertension," Larsen et al, 22nd European Meeting on Hypertension and Cardiovascular Protection. April 201

newspaper headlines summed it up: "As good as drugs". "The reduction in systolic blood pressure was quite significant – this is what powerful drugs do in trials," noted Glasgow University's Professor Anna Dominic-zak, the vice-president of the European Hypertension Society. "This is an initial study, so it needs to be confirmed, but it is potentially interesting as part of an overall strategy for managing hypertension in patients with low levels of vitamin D."[109]

The Koreans, meanwhile, have had more success linking arterial health with vitamin D in elderly patients. They didn't use cookies, so technically it wasn't a trial. They did however measure the arterial wall thickness of 1000 men and women over the age of 65 and selected randomly for a cohort study.

They found those with the lowest vitamin D levels (below 15 ng/ml) were three times more likely to have significant coronary artery stenosis than people with vitamin D levels higher than 30 ng/ml.[110]

Congestive heart disease, heart attacks and blood pressure are not the only areas where the sunshine vitamin is showing promise. It's being hailed as protective against fatal strokes as well.

---

[109]   "Vitamin D supplements 'as good as drugs' at reducing BP," *ZeeNews India*, 26 April 2012

[110]   "Vitamin D inadequacy is associated with significant coronary artery stenosis in a community based elderly cohort etc," Lim et al, *Journal of Endocrinology & Metabolism*, January 1, 2012, Vol. 97(1):169-178

A study of nearly 8,000 Americans found whites were more than twice as likely to suffer a fatal stroke if they have low vitamin D levels, defined in the study as less than 15 ng/ml, compared to a benchmark level of 31 ng/ml. Interestingly, the same effect was not found in African-Americans, even though they have proportionately more fatal strokes than Americans of European ancestry.

"Vitamin D deficiency was associated with an increased risk of stroke death in whites but not in blacks. Although blacks had a higher rate of fatal stroke compared with whites, the low 25(OH)D levels in blacks were unrelated to stroke incidence. Therefore 25(OH)D levels did not explain this excess risk."[111]

In Hawaii, the complete medical records of 8,000 Japanese-American men who'd visited the doctor in the mid 1960s as part of the Honolulu Heart Programme were examined to see how they'd fared over time. After ruling out those with pre-existing stroke conditions, the sample of just under 7,400 was studied for health outcomes up to and including the 1999 year – a 34 year timespan for those who'd first been enrolled in the study in 1965.[112]

---

111 "25-Hydroxyvitamin D deficiency is associated with fatal stroke among whites but not blacks: The NHANES-III linked mortality files," Michos et al, *Nutrition*, Volume 28, Issue 4, April 2012, Pages 367–371

112 "Low Dietary Vitamin D Predicts 34-Year Incident Stroke," Kojima et al, *Stroke*, first published online before print, May 2012, doi: 10.1161/STROKEAHA.112.651752

Of the 7,385 men, 960 went on to suffer strokes later in life. Based on the detailed dietary analysis provided during regular check-ups as part of the Heart Programme, researchers were able to calculate dietary intake of vitamin D.

Men with the lowest dietary intake of vitamin D were found to have had a 27% increased risk of ischemic stroke.

For women, the story might be even better.

The Harvard School of Public Health has recently published the findings of a meta-analysis of current research, where results from similar studies are pooled and examined to provide a larger dataset. Based on the comparison of 464 women who had experienced ischemic stroke, and a similar control group who hadn't, researchers found women with the highest levels of vitamin D reduced their risk of ischemic stroke by 49%.[113]

Further drilling down into a group of datasets, the Harvard team found women in the highest vitamin D group enjoyed up to 59% reduction in stroke risk. "Maintaining adequate vitamin D status may lower the risk of stroke in women," the study concluded.

In the long run, given that it's usually either heart disease or cancer that takes you in the end, the studies on longevity tell the biggest story.

---

113   "25-Hydroxyvitamin D Levels and the Risk of Stroke: A Prospective Study and Meta-analysis," Qi Sun et al, *Stroke*, Published online before print March 22, 2012, doi: 10.1161/ STROKEAHA.111.636910

When data from the blood samples of 3,400 Americans was analysed in the Third National Health And Nutrition Examination Survey (NHANES III), researchers found those with the lowest vitamin D levels were three times more likely to die of heart disease, and two and a half times more likely to die of any cause.[114] That's not a measure of absolute mortality, of course, because clearly we all die eventually, but cancer and heart disease are taking people early so if you can put it off for a while you reap the rewards.

More significantly from a community point of view, less disease means lower healthcare costs, and more productive time per capita.

A recently released study by the University of Washington further shatters the myth that there's no proof of a link between low vitamin D and tragedy. The research team wanted to find out how much vitamin D needed to be circulating in the blood to lower risk of serious events, and to do that they tested blood samples of 1,621 Caucasian adults.[115]

114   "Prospective Study of Serum 25-Hydroxyvitamin D Level, Cardiovascular Disease Mortality, and All-Cause Mortality in Older U.S. Adults," Adit A. Ginde MD, MPH,Robert Scragg MBBS, PhD, Robert S. Schwartz MD,   Carlos A. Camargo Jr. MD, DrPH, *Journal of the American Geriatrics Society*, Volume 57, Issue 9, pages 1595–1603, September 2009, http://onlinelibrary.wiley.com/doi/10.1111/j.1532-5415.2009.02359.x/full
115   "Serum 25-hydroxyvitamin D concentration and risk for major clinical disease events in a community-based population of older adults: a cohort study," de Boer et al, *Annals of Internal*

The samples had been in storage since the Cardiovascular Health Study of the early 1990s, and one of the great things about blood banks is that researchers can go back decades now in some cases and test samples. This particular test cohort had been aged 65 and over when their blood was first stored.

Having obtained their 25(OH)D blood serum readings, the research team then pulled out the medical files for each patient to discover what had happened to them. More to the point, they wanted to know how soon after the blood test the patient had suffered a "major event".

Of the 1,621 tested, within the next 11 years just over a thousand had indeed experienced an "event". The files revealed 335 developed cancer. A hundred and thirty-seven fractured a hip, 186 had heart attacks. Three hundred and sixty had died.

Study leader Ian de Boer told journalists that the likelihood of these "events" rose the lower the patient's vitamin D level was. There were strong seasonal signals, reflecting the low vitamin D generation during winter and spring, and the high vitamin D levels of summer and autumn.

Significantly, the danger point was when blood serum levels of vitamin D fell below 20 ng/ml (50 nmol/L), which is lower than the 30 ng/ml threshold most vitamin D experts now recognise.

Medicine, 2012 May 1;156(9):627-34

What's important to remember is that nearly every vitamin D study has identified a sliding scale where the benefits become more pronounced the closer the patient gets to 40 or 50 ng/ml (100 to 125 nmol/L). But sliding scales mean a trend can be identified early, at 20 ng/ml for example, whilst allowing that benefits would likely be greater and the trend even stronger if blood levels were even higher. Statistical probability curves allow for the fact that while some people will start seeing benefits at lower levels, a greater number will join that trend further up the scale.

One of the things to emerge from ongoing research, however, is that simply popping a vitamin D pill will not necessarily bring results. Case in point: a study of 107,811 people in the US found those with vitamin D levels higher than 30 ng/ml had a "statistically significant" lower risk with their lipid levels [fats in the blood]. This much we know. Researchers then wondered whether giving vitamin deficient patients a D supplement to improve their vitamin D blood levels would have a flow on effect and improve their lipids.

They tried. It didn't.

A sub-sample of 8,592 patients were given supplements, which did indeed raise their 25(OH)D serum levels, but which did not have any major impact over the 26 week study on LDL cholesterol or triglycerides. There was a small impact on HDL cholesterol for these patients.

"The seemingly conflicting findings of the cross-sectional analysis and longitudinal analysis suggest that while vitamin D deficiency is associated with an unfavorable lipid profile, correcting a deficiency through therapeutic vitamin D supplementation may have limited value in improving lipids," study leader Manish Ponda told journalists.[116]

In this case, he suspects, the vitamin D, rather than causing improved lipid profiles, may simply reflect better lipid profiles in those patients.

For participants in one recent study, however, vitamin D has been good news. Three thousand patients with heart failure were measured against a 47,000 control group. Those with the highest vitamin D levels, in both the sample and the controls, had the lowest risk of dying. And on the subject of popping pills, heart failure patients taking pills reduced their future mortality risk by 32%.[117]

That's got to be worth something to someone, somewhere.

116   http://www.sacbee.com/2012/07/17/4637302/vitamin-d-supplementation-may.html
117   "Vitamin D deficiency is a predictor of reduced survival in patients with heart failure; vitamin D supplementation improves outcome," Gotsman et al, *European Journal of Heart Failure*, 2012, doi: 10.1093/eurjhf/hfr175

Chapter 8

COMMON INFECTIONS

"Whether vitamin D should be implemented as a mandatory vitamin to prevent pandemic influenza is the question"

– *Journal of Medical Hypotheses, 2010*

There's an often repeated saying, "there's no cure for the common cold". It's not entirely true anymore – scientists have recently discovered an essential extract from a little-known South African geranium with the unpronounceable name "umckaloaba" has unique anti-bacterial and anti-viral properties that allow it to knock colds, common influenza, pneumonia and bronchitis on the head. They had to give it a more user friendly name – Kaloba – and it's now registered in several countries including Australia as a medicine because of its success in clinical trials.[118]

---

118   It's also proven successful at doing the unthinkable – killing the herpes virus in topical application in lab tests. See *Investigate* magazine, Jun/Jul 2012 issue, http://www.investigatedaily.com

The thing about Kaloba is that it actually stimulates the body's immune system into responding more powerfully and swiftly to incoming infections. Intriguingly, that's what vitamin D appears to do as well.

While vitamin D might not give you relief from a cold in three days, like Kaloba, there are studies that indicate people with high vitamin D levels get far fewer colds and infections in the first place.

A randomized controlled trial published in 2007 tested three groups for a year. One group received a capsule containing 2000IU of vitamin D to be taken each day. The second group received a capsule containing an 800IU daily dose, and the third received a placebo.[119]

Nearly all of those taking the placebo were found to have suffered colds or influenza during the year-long trial. Only one person taking the 2000IU daily supplement reported cold/influenza symptoms. Remember, none of the participants knew whether they were in the vitamin D group or not.

The people taking the lower dose 800IU supplement reported some cold/flu symptoms, but an order of magnitude fewer than those on the placebo.

What appears to be important however is not the size of the supplement itself, but how long you've been taking it and whether your blood levels of vitamin D

---

119   "Epidemic influenza and vitamin D," Aloia & Li-Ng, Epidemiol Infect 2007; 135:1095-1096

have been brought up to a protective level.

A second trial by the same research team two years later tested 162 adults in a randomised trial over the 12 weeks of the winter season. Half the sample received 2000IU a day, and the other half a placebo.[120]

Unlike their first year long study, this one beginning at the start of winter showed no protective effect of vitamin D at all. Why would that be? Possibly because at the start of winter your vitamin D levels have already fallen below par in most cases, so you are starting from a catch-up rather than optimum position.

The previous study actually had a twist in the tale that proves the point I am making. Although reported as a "year long trial", it had actually begun as a three year trial. For the first two years, the vitamin D participants had been receiving only the 800IU dose. Then in the final year they boosted the dosage for some of those people to 2000IU and commenced a year long drag race to the finish. This meant that many of those with the high-dose vitamin D had actually been taking vitamin D for three years, giving them a chance to seriously lock in the blood serum benefits.

Placed in perspective, it's not hard to see why the second study over the 12 week winter season flopped.

---

120   "A randomized controlled trial of vitamin D3 supplementation for the prevention of symptomatic upper respiratory tract infections," Li-Ng et al, *Epidemiol. Infect.* (2009), 137, 1396–1404.

The secret is really in the long-term blood levels, not the size of the daily supplement.

Which is exactly the conclusion the researchers reached in regard to their second study:

"There are several reasons why vitamin D3 supplementation may have been ineffective at preventing URIs [upper respiratory tract infections] in this study. First, the subjects started vitamin D3 supplementation during the wintertime and not beforehand. It takes about 3 months for 25-OHD levels to reach a steady state with supplementation. Because it takes a significant amount of time to build up vitamin D stores, the effect of vitamin D supplementation lagged behind the cold and influenza season. Vitamin D3 supplementation may be more effective in preventing URIs if started during autumn when sunlight begins to decrease."

Other reasons include that the people in the first 2007 study began with much lower vitamin D levels (18.4 ng/ml average), meaning the control group remained vitamin D deficient while the vitamin takers improved. In the second 2009 study, however, both controls and vitamin-takers began with an average baseline of 25.6 ng/ml, meaning they were both already out of the danger zone.

Proof of this thesis can be seen in the actual rates of infection. In the 2007 study, 30 of the 39 placebo-takers reported a URI (77%). In the 2009 study only 41%

of those on placebo suffered an infection. We know the placebo-takers had much higher vitamin D blood levels than those in the first study, and they suffered a big drop in reported infections. Ergo, point proved.

Another randomised, double-blind trial conducted at Yale University involving nearly 200 people in 2010 has gone on to prove that people with low vitamin D levels are twice as likely to develop respiratory tract infections:

"One hundred ninety-five (98.5%) of the enrolled participants completed the study. Light skin pigmentation, lean body mass, and supplementation with vitamin D were found to correlate with higher concentrations of 25-hydroxyvitamin D. Concentrations of 38 ng/ml or more were associated with a significant (p<0.0001) two-fold reduction in the risk of developing acute respiratory tract infections and with a marked reduction in the percentages of days ill."[121]

The inferences to be drawn from this are obvious, they say:

"Maintenance of a 25-hydroxyvitamin D serum concentration of 38 ng/ml or higher should significantly reduce the incidence of acute viral respiratory tract infections and the burden of illness caused thereby, at least during the fall and winter in temperate zones.

---

121   "Serum 25-Hydroxyvitamin D and the Incidence of Acute Viral Respiratory Tract Infections in Healthy Adults," Sabetta et al, *PLoS ONE* 5(6): e11088. doi:10.1371/journal.pone.0011088

The findings of the present study provide direction for and call for future interventional studies examining the efficacy of vitamin D supplementation in reducing the incidence and severity of specific viral infections, including influenza, in the general population and in subpopulations with lower 25-hydroxyvitamin D concentrations, such as pregnant women, dark skinned individuals, and the obese."

So the sunshine vitamin substantially reduces your family's risk of catching colds or flu – who knew?

We've touched on possible reasons for this in earlier chapters but it's worth another look. Vitamin D is known to stimulate the immune system into producing natural antibiotics, as Li-Ng's 2009 study explains:[122]

"The active form of vitamin D, 1,25-dihydroxyvitamin D (1,25-OH2D) increases the production of endogenous [it means self-made naturally] antibiotics called antimicrobial peptides (AMP).[123]

"AMPs such as defensin and cathelicidin have a broad range of actions against microorganisms, including bacteria, fungi and viruses. Defensins can block viral infection by directly acting on the virion or by affect-

---

122　"A randomized controlled trial of vitamin D3 supplementation for the prevention of symptomatic upper respiratory tract infections," Li-Ng et al, *Epidemiol. Infect.* (2009), 137, 1396–1404 http://www.vitaminedelft.org/files/art/ling2009.pdf
123　"Cutting edge: 1,25-dihydroxyvitamin D3 is a direct inducer of antimicrobial peptide gene expression," Wang TT, et al. *Journal of Immunology* 2004; 173: 2909–2912.

ing the target cell and thereby indirectly interfering with viral infection.[124] One of the defensins called retrocyclin-2 inhibits influenza virus infection."[125]

It's yet more proof that dermatologists are fundamentally and dangerously wrong when they tell us to "avoid the sun...there is no safe level of exposure". Our bodies are designed to interact with sunlight to create antibiotics and antivirals. Over the past century, and in particular the past fifty years, we have moved away from our natural place under the sun, and we are reaping the rewards of that decision healthwise.

While US regulators um and ah over vitamin D, the European Food Safety Authority has ruled that the compound is immunoprotective:[126]

"The Panel concludes that a cause and effect relationship has been established between the dietary intake of vitamin D and contribution to the normal function of the immune system and healthy inflammatory response, and maintenance of normal muscle function."

124   "Defensins in innate antiviral immunity," Klotman ME, Chang TL. *Nature Reviews Immunology* 2006; 6: 447–456.

125   "Carbohydrate-binding molecules inhibit viral fusion and entry by crosslinking membrane glycoproteins," Leikina E, et al. *Nature Immunology* 2005; 6: 995–1001

126   The panel also ruled that vitamin D's impact on cardiovascular health had not been sufficiently proven, but at the time of the ruling they did not have the benefit of the recent studies I've included in this book in the cardio chapter. *EFSA Journal* 2010; 8(2):1468 [17 pp.]. doi:10.2903/j.efsa.2010.1468

Even as they announced that, the scientific test results continued to roll in.

A Japanese research team managed to stave off Influenza A in schoolchildren in a randomized trial of vitamin D supplements. Three hundred and thirty four children were split into groups receiving either 1200IU of vitamin D a day, or a placebo.

The test ran through the northern hemisphere winter, from December 2008 through March 2009, and overall children on supplements reduced their risk of infection by 42% compared with children in the control group. As reported earlier in this book, the improvement was even more significant for children with a history of asthma – they slashed their risk of influenza A by 83%.[127]

The impact of vitamin D levels on influenza risk is leading to some researchers openly discussing whether vitamin D supplementation should be a mandatory public health step in preparation for the next global flu pandemic:[128]

"Influenza was associated with a higher tendency

---

127   "Randomized trial of vitamin D supplementation to prevent seasonal Influenza A in schoolchildren," Urashima et al, *American Journal of Clinical Nutrition*, 2010, May, 91(5):1255-60
128   "Vitamin D's potential to reduce the risk of hospital-acquired infections," Youssef et al, *Dermato-Endocrinology*, Volume 4, Issue 2 April/May/June 2012, http://www.landesbioscience.com/journals/dermatoendocrinology/article/20789/?show_full_text=true&

to develop superimposed bacterial pneumonia, and prevention may avoid the higher risk of pneumonia, especially in elderly and chronic lung disease patients. Whether vitamin D should be implemented as a mandatory vitamin to prevent pandemic influenza is the question.[129] Juzeniene et al. studied pandemic and non-pandemic influenzas in Sweden, Norway, the United States, Singapore, and Japan. The higher exposure to UVB radiation in summer and consequently higher 25(OH)D levels protect against influenza.[130]

It's not just colds and flu that vitamin D has been proven to help protect you against.

TUBERCULOSIS

One of the classic infections it helps beat is tuberculosis, a disease that's been preying on humans since the dawn of time. Characterised by the disintegration of lung tissue to the point of fatality, and easily spread by contact and coughing, it's a vicious disease that, coincidentally is re-emerging in the population in much the same way that rickets is back in the news.

"There is no need to get vaccinated against tuberculo-

129   "Pandemic influenza A (H1N1): mandatory vitamin D supplementation?" Goldstein et al. *Med Hypotheses* 2010; 74:756; PMID: 20006449; DOI: 10.1016/j.mehy.2009.11.006

130   "The seasonality of pandemic and non-pandemic influenzas: the roles of solar radiation and vitamin D," Juzeniene et al, *Int J Infect Dis* 2010; 14:e1099-105; PMID: 21036090; DOI: 10.1016/j. ijid.2010.09.002.

sis," reported *NaturalNews* recently,[131] "if you maintain high enough levels of vitamin D, suggests a new study published in the journal *Science Translational Medicine*. Researchers found that, in the presence of even minimally adequate levels of vitamin D, the body's own immune system will naturally trigger an immune response against the disease and many others without the need for drug or chemical interventions."

The real lesson to take from this is not that tuberculosis is beating modern antibiotics because of increased antibiotic resistance. No, the real lesson is that you are only likely to contract tuberculosis in the first place if your vitamin D levels are low.

Often, the disease strikes in Africa and Asia. A recent Pakistani study found people with low vitamin D levels were 500% more likely to fall victim to tuberculosis. You might assume that being relatively sunny in Pakistan they'd be OK, but in truth most people, particularly women, are fully clothed from head to toe. Those surveyed had vitamin D levels as low as 4.6 ng/ml, a sharp contrast with the ideal target of between 40 and 50 ng/ml.

"In this cohort follow-up study from Pakistan," concluded the researchers, "low vitamin D levels were associated with progression to active TB disease in healthy household contacts. No deaths occurred during the follow-up period from either TB or unrelated

---

131   http://www.naturalnews.com/033989_vitamin_D_
tuberculosis.html#ixzz217RYbqP7

causes. Our findings also suggest that vitamin D deficiency may explain the higher susceptibility of women to disease progression in our cohort."[132]

Similar low vitamin D levels were seen in Mongolian children, and vitamin D supplementation cut their risks of tuberculosis by 60%.[133]

It's that study from the journal *Science Translational Medicine*, however, that nails just how crucial vitamin D is. They point out that combating TB worldwide depends on understanding how human immune systems work to fight infections.

"Acquired T cell responses are critical for host defense against microbial pathogens, yet the mechanisms by which they act in humans remain unclear," reports lead author Mario Fabri.[134]

It is said that 'sunlight is the best disinfectant', and that's exactly what Fabri's team discovered. They found that T-cells are fired up with interferon and natural antibiotics like cathelicidin to batter Mycobacterium tuberculosis when it infects the human body. Without

132   "Vitamin D Deficiency and Tuberculosis Progression," Talat et al, *Emerging Infectious Diseases*, Volume 16, Number 5 – May 2010, http://wwwnc.cdc.gov/eid/article/16/5/09-1693.htm

133   "Vitamin D, tuberculin skin test conversion, and latent tuberculosis in Mongolian school-age children: a randomized, double-blind, placebo-controlled feasibility trial," Ganmaa et al, *Am J Clin Nutr* August 2012 ajcn.034967

134   "Vitamin D Is Required for IFN-y–Mediated Antimicrobial Activity of Human Macrophages," Fabri et al, *Sci Transl Med* 12 October 2011: Vol. 3, Issue 104, p. 104ra102

vitamin D to ignite the immune system, our biological engine coughs a couple of times and gives up, becoming overwhelmed with the infection.

Fabri's researchers discovered something else as well. Dark-skinned people are more vulnerable to diseases like TB because of genetic variations that are preventing them from manufacturing sufficient amounts of vitamin D. That deficiency was able to be rectified through supplements.

"These results suggest a mechanism in which vitamin D is required for acquired immunity to overcome the ability of intracellular pathogens to evade macrophage-mediated antimicrobial responses. The present findings underscore the importance of adequate amounts of vitamin D in all human populations for sustaining both innate and acquired immunity against infection."

HOSPITAL SUPERBUGS

In the western world, hospital-acquired infections – diseases you pick up during a stay in hospital – are actually the biggest cause of death in the health system. Nearly two million cases are reported each year in US hospitals alone, and 100,000 deaths are attributable to them each year in the United States.

A review published 2012 reveals the costs of these avoidable infections to US consumers alone are up to $45 billion a year.[135]

---

135   "Vitamin D's potential to reduce the risk of hospital-

"Health care–associated and hospital-acquired infections are two entities associated with increased morbidity and mortality. They are highly costly and constitute a great burden to the health care system. Vitamin D deficiency (< 20 ng/ml) is prevalent and may be a key contributor to both acute and chronic ill health. Vitamin D deficiency is associated with decreased innate immunity and increased risk for infections. Vitamin D can positively influence a wide variety of microbial infections."

In terms of what you are likely to catch in hospital, "Pneumonia was the most likely disease, followed by bacteremias, urinary tract infections, surgical site infections, and others."

Nearly 13% – or roughly one in eight – people admitted to American hospitals end up with one of these infections, prolonging their stay in hospital or sometimes killing them. The latest study pegs the cost of treating these people at up to US$21,000 per person, with an extra US$33,000 loading per infectee across the board in the costs associated with premature death and lost earning potential for the percentage who die. That's up to $54,000 on average, per person. Little wonder health administrators are trying to find ways to reduce the risk.

---

acquired infections," Youssef et al, *Dermato-Endocrinology,* Volume 4, Issue 2 April/May/June 2012, http://www.landesbioscience. com/journals/dermatoendocrinology/article/20789/?show_full_ text=true&

The new review says the answer probably lies with vitamin D:

"Vitamin D modulates the immune system[136] and appears to have systemic antimicrobial effects[137] that may be crucial in a variety of both acute and chronic illness.

"In a previous publication, we outlined the most important actions of vitamin D against many infections, whether they are bacterial, mycobacterial, fungal, parasitic, or viral.[138] We also found that vitamin D deficiency was intimately linked to adverse health outcomes and costs in veterans with staphylococcal and *Clostridium difficile(C. difficile)* infections. Vitamin D–deficient patients with *C. difficile* or staphylococcal infections had costs more than five times higher than those of nondeficient patients. The total length of hospital stay was four times greater in the vitamin D–deficient group. Also, the total number of hospitalizations was significantly greater in vitamin D–deficient patients.[139]

136   [Studies on the antimicrobial effect of vitamin D (author's transl)]. Feindt E, Ströder J. Klin Wochenschr 1977; 55:507-8; PMID: 195120; DOI: 10.1007/BF01489010

137   "The role of vitamin D in regulating immune responses," Toubi & Shoenfeld, *Isr Med Assoc J* 2010; 12:174-5; PMID: 20684184

138   "Antimicrobial implications of vitamin D," Youssef et al. *Dermato-Endocrinol* 2011; 3:1-10; PMID: 21519401; DOI: 10.4161/derm.3.4.15027

139   "Healthcare costs of Staphylococcus aureus and Clostridium

"Similarly, vitamin D–deficient patients with MRSA and *Pseudomonas aeruginosa* infections had higher costs and service utilization than patients who were not vitamin D deficient.[140] In a retrospective study by McKinney and colleagues, ICU survivors had a significantly lower rate of vitamin D deficiency than did nonsurvivors (28% vs. 53%). The risk of death was significantly higher in ICU patients with vitamin D deficiency.[141]

The study reports that one Seattle surgeon specialising in treating war veterans has taken to routinely giving patients a 50,000IU dose of vitamin D before surgery, and found that post-surgery complications have almost disappeared. It's an issue being looked at in intensive care units as well.

One study of ICU patients found 82% were either vitamin D deficient or insufficient. Those with optimal vitamin D were more likely to recover and go home soonest. Those at the lowest levels of vitamin D were

---

difficile infections in veterans: role of vitamin D deficiency," Youssef et al. *Epidemiol Infect* 2010; 138:1322-7; PMID: 20056018; DOI: 10.1017/S0950268809991543.

140   "Healthcare costs of methicillin resistant Staphylococcus aureus and Pseudomonas aeruginosa infections in veterans: role of vitamin D deficiency," Youssef et al. *Eur J Clin Microbiol Infect Dis* 2012; 31:281-6; PMID: 21695580; DOI: 10.1007/s10096-011-1308-9

141   "Relationship between vitamin D status and ICU outcomes in veterans," McKinney et al. *J Am Med Dir Assoc* 2011; 12:208-11; PMID: 21333923; DOI: 10.1016/j.jamda.2010.04.004

more likely to catch an infection and stay longer.[142]

"Vitamin D therefore appears to be important for patients with critical illness."

An Israeli research team discovered that the lives of patients admitted to intensive care units and placed on mechanical life support in that country literally depended on their vitamin D levels. Those with the lowest levels were more likely to die, and die sooner. Of the 130 critical care patients studied, those with the highest vitamin D levels lived longer in the ICU and had better levels of white blood cells to fight infection.

The study examined blood vitamin D levels on admission. A hundred and seven of the patients were deficient, with an average of less than 15 ng/ml. The study looked at their survival rates up to sixty days. Of the 44% who died, those with the lowest vitamin D levels lasted only 15 days on average, whereas those who had been admitted with higher vitamin D levels lived for 24 days and their bodies showed more signs of fighting to live.[143]

And what of our love hate relationship with antibiotics?

"Currently, prescribing traditional antimicrobials

142   "Relationship of Vitamin D Deficiency to Clinical Outcomes in Critically Ill Patients," Higgins et al, JPEN *J Parenter Enteral Nutr* 2012; ; PMID: 22523178; DOI: 10.1177/0148607112444449

143   "Vitamin D deficiency is associated with poor outcomes and increased mortality in severely ill patients," Arnson et al, *QJM,* (2012) doi: 10.1093/qjmed/hcs014

for infectious processes is customary in medicine. The current use of antimicrobials in the United States costs billions of dollars, and the overuse of antibiotics persists and contributes to the emergence of resistant organisms. Vitamin D is likely to emerge as a powerful and hitherto unrecognized antimicrobial agent. Evidence is mounting that vitamin D could help to manage infectious illnesses."[144]

To get the jump on superbug infections, however, doesn't come easy. The research team recommended vitamin D blood levels of at least 95 nmol/L (38 ng/ml) to boost immunity enough to achieve a 50% risk reduction in MRSA infection.

Once again, the over-riding message: boost your vitamin D levels before you actually need them in a crisis. It may be the difference between life and death.

---

144 "Vitamin D's potential to reduce the risk of hospital-acquired infections," Youssef et al, Dermato-Endocrinology, Volume 4, Issue 2 April/May/June 2012, http://www.landesbioscience.com/journals/dermatoendocrinology/article/20789/?show_full_text=true&

Chapter 9

CONCEPTION, PREGNANCY, CHILDHOOD: WHY YOUR BABY NEEDS VITAMIN D

"Our statistics suggest that it could explain about 40 percent of all schizophrenias. That's a much bigger effect than we're used to seeing in schizophrenia research"

– John McGrath, Queensland Brain Institute, 2010

You've probably heard the radio ads for erectile dysfunction. For men, it's a little like those ads from the sixties and seventies where the skinny weakling on the beach gets sand kicked in his face by a musclebound Adonis. The latter may have been pitching a bodybuilding programme, but the psychology behind the advertising is the same.

The moral of erectile dysfunction, however, appears to be that if the skinny weakling had spent more time sunbathing he'd probably be fine in the sack. From our 'not-that-as-well?' file comes the news that the sunshine vitamin has been linked to sexual performance issues.

The logic behind it is laid out in a recent report in the medical journal Dermato-Endocrinology, which points out that half of ED cases are caused by vascular health issues. With vitamin D's role in maintaining the cardiovascular system and keeping blood pumping to the extremities, researchers say getting a vitamin D check-up is probably a wise idea.

"The treatment of choice for ED has been the use of phosphodiesterase-5 inhibitors such as Viagra," says study author Marc Sorenson.

"While effective in relieving the ED symptoms, these drugs do nothing for the underlying cause and may lose their effectiveness over time. They may also hide from users the possibility of cardiovascular disease...if proven in further research, vitamin D optimization has the potential to influence the cause of ED to prevent or mitigate the condition."

It may sound like something to chortle over, but Sorenson says it's actually deadly serious. When erectile dysfunction appears, it can sometimes be a harbinger of something much worse.

"Although nonvascular factors such as depression, fatigue, stress, Parkinson disease, multiple sclerosis (MS), and hypertensive medications may affect ED,[145]

---

145   "Erectile dysfunction and the cardiovascular patient: endothelial dysfunction is the common denominator," Solomon et al. *Heart* 2003; 89:251-3; PMID: 12591819; DOI: 10.1136/heart.89.3.251.

it is primarily a vasculogenic disease. Its most prevalent cause is the arterial occlusion of atherosclerosis, which also affects the coronary arteries and can lead to heart attack[146] or, in other parts of the body, vascular events such as stroke[147] and peripheral arterial disease (PAD).[148]"

For all the reasons that you would take vitamin D to help maintain heart and cardiovascular health, the benefits of doing so might actually help you dodge an appointment down the track with an erectile dysfunction specialist.

Apart from affecting your ability to sexually perform, vitamin D turns out to have other fundamental roles in conception: creating healthy sperm[149] and boosting the fertility[150] and sexual health of both men and

146   "Erectile dysfunction as a harbinger for increased cardiometabolic risk," Billups et al, *Int J Impot Res* 2008; 20:236-42; PMID: 18200018; DOI: 10.1038/sj.ijir.3901634.

147   "Aortic atherosclerotic disease and stroke," Kronzon I, Tunick PA. *Circulation* 2006; 114:63-75; PMID: 16818829; DOI: 10.1161/CIRCULATIONAHA.105.593418

148   Stöppler MC, Lee D, Kulic D, Peripheral MD. Vascular Disease. *MedicineNet.com*. http://www.medicinenet.com/peripheral_vascular_disease/article.htm

149   "Vitamin D is positively associated with sperm motility and increases intracellular calcium in human spermatozoa," Jensen et al, *Human Reproduction* (2011) 26 (6): 1307-1317. doi: 10.1093/humrep/der059

150   "Circulating vitamin D correlates with serum antimüllerian hormone levels in late-reproductive-aged women: Women's Interagency HIV Study", Mehri et al, *Fertility and Sterility*, Volume 98, Issue 1 , Pages 228-234, July 2012

women[151]. Vitamin D has been linked to higher tes-tosterone and androgen levels in men,[152] and is heavily linked to women's reproductive health.

"There is some evidence, that in addition to sex ste-roid hormones, the classic regulators of reproduction, vitamin D also modulates reproductive processes in women and men," say the research team behind one recent analysis.[153]

Around 15% of couples report fertility problems, and 30-40% of those are related to male issues including sperm quality. Again, it's no surprise to see fertility problems rising in the wake of two decades of slip, slop, slap sun avoidance messages.

In women, vitamin D – which is in reality a steroid hormone – lowers the dominance of estrogen, thereby helping improve fertility as well as lowering breast cancer risk.[154] On the other hand, low vitamin D levels

151   "Vitamin D metabolism, sex hormones and male reproductive function," Jensen, M, *Reproduction* May 25, 2012 REP-12-0064
152   Wehr E, Pilz S, Boehm BO, März W, Obermayer-Pietsch B. Association of vitamin D status with serum androgen levels in men. *Clin Endocrinol*(Oxf), 2009 Dec 29.
153   "Vitamin D and fertility – a systematic review," Elisabeth Lerchbaum and Barbara Obermayer-Pietsch, *Eur J Endocrinol.* 2012 May;166(5):765-78. Epub 2012 Jan 24, http://www.eje-online.org/content/early/2012/01/24/EJE-11-0984.full.pdf
154   "Vitamin D association with estradiol and progesterone in young women," Knight et al, *Cancer Causes & Control.* 2010 Mar;21(3):479-83

appear to be strongly associated with infertility, as a team from Yale University discovered in 2008:

"Of note, not a single patient with either ovulatory disturbance or polycystic ovary syndrome demonstrated normal Vitamin D levels; 39 per cent of those with ovulatory disturbance and 38 per cent of those with PCOS had serum 25OHD levels consistent with deficiency," Yale's Dr Lubna Pal told journalists.[155]

"Given the pandemic of Vitamin D insufficiency, if indeed our observations are substantiated, aggressive repletion with Vitamin D may emerge as an alternative approach to facilitate ovulation resumption with minimal to no risk for ovarian hyperstimulation syndrome or multiple pregnancy."

A staggering 93% of infertile women treated by the Yale team were either clinically deficient or insufficient in vitamin D.

Fertility forums on the internet are rife with women who haven't been able to get pregnant and whose obstetricians are now prescribing megadoses of vitamin D (50,000IU a week for several weeks) to improve their blood levels and chances of healthy conception.

Low vitamin D levels may be linked to second trimester miscarriage.[156]

155   "Vitamin D can aid fertility," by Rebecca Smith, *The Telegraph*, 11 November 2008
156   "Effects of 25OHD concentrations on chances of pregnancy and pregnancy outcomes: a cohort study in healthy Danish women," Mølle et al, *European Journal of Clinical Nutrition* (2012) 66, 862–

It is, however, in pregnancy itself that vitamin D is so crucial, and at levels far above those contained in pregnancy multivitamins: "During pregnancy, supplementation with the current standard amount of vitamin D in prenatal vitamins – 400 IU (10 µg) vitamin D/day – has minimal effect on circulating 25(OH)D concentrations in the mother and her infant."[157]

"There is considerable evidence that low maternal levels of 25 hydroxyvitamin D are associated with adverse outcomes for both mother and fetus in pregnancy as well as the neonate and child.[158]

"Vitamin D deficiency during pregnancy has been linked with a number of maternal problems including infertility, preeclampsia, gestational diabetes and an increased rate of caesarean section.

"Likewise, for the child, there is an association with small size, impaired growth and skeletal problems in infancy, neonatal hypocalcaemia and seizures, and an increased risk of HIV transmission. Other childhood disease associations include type 1 diabetes and effects on immune tolerance."

You can add childhood obesity to that list. Over

868; doi:10.1038/ejcn.2012.18

157   "Vitamin D and Its Role During Pregnancy in Attaining Optimal Health of Mother and Fetus," Wagner et al, *Nutrients* 2012, 4(3), 208-230; doi:10.3390/nu4030208

158   "Vitamin D and pregnancy: An old problem revisited," Barrett H, McElduff A, *Best Practice & Research, Clinical Endocrinology & Metabolism.* 2010 Aug;24(4):527-39.

the past thirty years, we've increasingly become fatter. Now a new study is blaming part of that on low vitamin D during pregnancy.

Researchers at the University of Southampton followed up the pregnancy blood samples of 977 women by comparing them to the health outcomes of their children by age 6. Low vitamin D levels in mothers were found to result in lower weight babies, but ironically fatter children by the age of six, even after controlling for lifestyle, physical activity, body mass index and other factors.[159]

It is too early to know how, but researchers believe there is something about vitamin D that helps lock in fat regulation mechanisms in the developing foetus. [160] Further possible evidence of this emerged in another recent study of seriously obese teenagers undergoing bariatric surgery. Fifty-four percent were either deficient or severely deficient in vitamin D, and although obese people are routinely low in vitamin D, in this case race played a huge part. Eighty-two percent of

159   "Maternal vitamin D status in pregnancy is associated with adiposity in the offspring," Crozier et al, *American Journal of Clinical Nutrition*, July 2012, doi: 10.3945/ajcn.112.037473
160   It may also help adults. A study of women over 65 in the USA found those with lower vitamin D levels had a higher weight gain over the four and a half year trial. See "Associations Between 25-Hydroxyvitamin D and Weight Gain in Elderly Women," LeBlanc et al, *Journal of Women's Health*, online 25 June 2012, doi:10.1089/jwh.2012.3506

African-American teens in the study were deficient or worse, 59% of Hispanics and 37% of European-Americans.

"The US adolescent obesity rate has more than tripled in the past 30 years," reported one medical journal on the study, "with 16% of children and adolescents now overweight, 4% obese and 4% morbidly obese."[161]

As we discussed in the Asthma chapter, mothers with low vitamin D levels during pregnancy are more likely to have children with asthma and/or common allergies. Children with 25(OH)D levels lower than 15 ng/ml are a whopping 240% more likely to have a peanut allergy than children with 30 ng/ml vitamin D, for example.[162] Another case-control study in 2012 reported children with low vitamin D levels in their first year of life are almost four times more likely to develop food allergies.[163]

A comprehensive review of vitamin D in pregnancy published recently, and available to read in full on the

161   "Check vitamin D in adolescents before bariatric surgery," *Clinical Endocrinology News*, June 28 2012

162   "Vitamin D levels and food and environmental allergies in the United States: Results from the National Health and Nutrition Examination Survey 2005-2006," Sharief et al, *Journal of Allergy and Clinical Immunology*, Volume 127, Issue 5, May 2011, Pages 1195–1202

163   "Food allergic infants more likely to have vitamin D insufficiency," *Family Practice News*, 22 March 2012, citing Journal of Allergy and Clinical Immunology, 2012; 129[suppl.]:AB141

internet,[164] shows just how widespread deficiency in pregnancy is:

"Reports of profound [severe] deficiency among pregnant women, those with 25(OH)D concentrations <10 ng/mL (25 nmol/L) are common throughout the world: 18% of pregnant women studied in the UK[165], 25% in the UAE ,[166] 80% in Iran,[167] 42% in northern India,[168] 61% in New Zealand ,[169] 89.5% in Japan,[170] and 60–84% of pregnant non-Western women in The Hague, Netherlands[171] had serum 25(OH)D concentrations <10 ng/mL (25 nmol/L).

164   "Vitamin D and Its Role During Pregnancy in Attaining Optimal Health of Mother and Fetus," Wagner et al, *Nutrients* 2012, 4(3), 208-230; doi:10.3390/nu4030208

165   "Maternal vitamin D status during pregancy and childhood bone mass at 9 years: A longitudinal study", Javaid et al. *Lancet* 2006, 367, 36-43

166   "Serum 25-hydroxyvitamin D and calcium homeostasis in the United Arab Emirates mothers and neonates: A preliminary report," Dawodu et al. *Middle East Paediatr.* 1997, 2, 9-12

167   "Vitamin D deficiency in Iranian mothers and their neonates: A pilot study," Bassir et al. *Acta Paediatr.* 2001, 90, 577-579

168   "High prevalence of vitamin D deficiency among pregnant women and their newborns in northern India," Sachan et al, *Am. J. Clin. Nutr.* 2005, 81, 1060-1064

169   "Vitamin D deficiency in pregnant New Zealand women," Judkins, A.; Eagleton, C.. *N. Z. Med. J.* 2006, 119, U2144

170   High prevalence of hypovitaminosis D in pregnant Japanese women with threatened premature delivery," Shibata et al. *J. Bone Miner. Metab.* 2011, 29, 615-620

171   "High prevalence of vitamin D deficiency in pregnant non-Western women the The Hague, Netherlands," Van der Meer et al. *Am. J. Clin. Nutr.* 2006, 84, 350-353

"Interestingly, in a recent study involving 144 pregnant women in the greater Copenhagen area evaluated at 18, 32 and 39 weeks of gestation, 1.4–4.3% had this degree of deficiency;[172] this lower rate may correlate with increased dietary intakes of fish. For those areas of the world with higher rates of deficiency, it appears that a long-standing unawareness of how vitamin D is made and of the short and long-term health consequences of vitamin D insufficiency has led to widespread insufficiencies in most populations."

New Zealand is one of the countries that has taken the sunsmart, slip, slop, slap message utterly to heart, and its 61% severe deficiency levels in pregnancy may be a direct result of educated New Zealand women avoiding the sun. Those levels would also explain the rise in rickets, autism, asthma, attention deficit disorder and some of the other conditions we're about to see.

Good levels of vitamin D are needed during pregnancy for proper development of your baby's skeleton, tooth enamel and growth and wellbeing. Women take folic acid to prevent neural tube defects in their babies like spina bifida, but with mothers hiding from the sun they're leaving their unborn children vulnerable to a range of other nasties.

Otherwise-healthy newborns, but with low vitamin

---

172   "Vitamin D status during normal pregnancy and postpartum. A longitudinal study in 141 Danish women," Milman et al. *J. Perinat. Med.* 2011, 40, 57-61

D levels, are six times more likely to fall victim to RSV, a virus responsible for the most serious lower respiratory tract bronchiolitis infections in infants.[173]

If a woman's vitamin D deficiency is severe whilst she is pregnant, she runs a heightened – albeit rare – risk that her baby may have hypocalcaemic seizures in the womb.

As we've already seen, a lack of vitamin D in pregnancy may lead to autism, and new research has added schizophrenia to that list. A 2010 study of 424 Danish schizophrenia sufferers matched them for both gender and birthdate with a control group of 424 people without the condition.

Using blood samples taken at birth and stored, researchers were able to look at the vitamin D levels of all the babies at birth. They discovered those babies with low levels of the vitamin were twice as likely to develop schizophrenia later in life.[174]

"Our statistics suggest that it could explain about 40 percent of all schizophrenias. That's a much bigger effect

173   "Cord Blood Vitamin D Deficiency Is Associated With Respiratory Syncytial Virus Bronchiolitis," Belderbos et al, *Pediatrics* Vol. 127 No. 6 June 1, 2011 pp. e1513 -e1520 (doi: 10.1542/peds.2010-3054), http://pediatrics.aappublications.org/content/127/6/e1513.full

174   "Neonatal Vitamin D Status and Risk of Schizophrenia – A Population-Based Case-Control Study," McGrath et al, *Arch Gen Psychiatry.* 2010;67(9):889-894. doi:10.1001/archgenpsychiatry.2010.110, http://archpsyc.jamanetwork.com/article.aspx?articleid=210878

than we're used to seeing in schizophrenia research," lead researcher John McGrath, of the Queensland Brain Institute in Australia, told reporters.[175]

There are other factors at play in schizophrenia, mainly genetic[176] and environmental,[177] but just as with autism it appears low vitamin D levels leave your child's body more vulnerable to whatever flicks the switch and brings those other factors into play.

There was a strange twist in the tail of this particular study, similar to the one discovered with that other Scandinavian study – the Finnish smokers. Just like that, the schizophrenia research team found that those with the absolute highest levels of vitamin D appeared to begin raising the risk again for schizophrenia. In statistical analysis, this is known as a "U-shaped curve",

---

175   "Low Vitamin D Linked to Schizophrenia," *Discovery News*, 7 Sep, 2010, http://news.discovery.com/human/vitamin-d-schizophrenia.html

176   If you are worried about possible mental illness in your children, have babies before the age of 25. Studies have shown a 17% increase in schizophrenia risk to children whose fathers are aged 30, rising to double the risk where Dad is 45, and three times the risk where Dad is aged over 50. The fault is thought to lie with spermatogenesis which, coincidentally, has been shown to improve in men with high vitamin D levels. "Advancing paternal age and the risk of schizophrenia," Malaspina et al, *Archives of General Psychiatry*, 2001 Apr;58(4):361-7

177   "The Antecedents of Schizophrenia: A Review of Birth Cohort Studies," Welham et al, *Schizophrenia Bulletin (2009) 35 (3): 603-623. doi: 10.1093/schbul/sbn084* http://schizophreniabulletin.oxfordjournals.org/content/35/3/603.full#ref-77

inasmuch if you follow the U, the risk goes down, then goes back up at some point.

The researchers on the Danish data haven't been able to find out why it happened, but they suspect it may be a genetic variation in the Scandinavian sample, where a certain number of people can have high circulating vitamin D in their blood, but a mutation prevents them from converting the vitamin in the blood to the biologically-active form of vitamin D actually used by the organs. In other words, their vitamin D processing system is not working properly – they have a lot of vitamin in the tank but the outflow pipe is blocked. They would appear in the sample with high levels of the vitamin, but wouldn't be getting the benefit of it, which could explain the apparent rising risk.[178]

---

178   This Scandinavian discrepancy, which is at odds with studies in other parts of the world, keeps popping up. In a study published August 2012, blood samples from 247,000 Danish citizens were analysed for mortality risk relative to vitamin D. The safest vitamin D levels for Danes appear to be 50-60 nmol/L (20-24 ng/ml). Compared with that bracket, Danes with lower vitamin D levels were 2.1 times more likely to have died, while that U-curve was back with the revelation that Danes with blood vitamin D levels higher than 140 nmol/L (56 ng/ml) were 1.4 times more likely to have died. For Scandinavians, the question has to be asked whether centuries of living in low vitamin D areas has caused micro-evolutionary responses. Are they, for example, more efficient at processing low levels of vitamin D, so that they're getting more bang from their D buck and don't need higher levels, or are they less efficient at processing, leaving high serum levels but less biologically-active vitamin D? See "A reverse J-shaped

It is a cautionary development, however, and all the more reason to get your vitamin D levels regularly checked by your doctor during pregnancy to ensure you are neither low nor excessively high. Because baby's skeleton is formed by stripping back minerals from a mother's bones, a lot of the vitamin D taken by a pregnant woman will be used to help replenish and rebuild, in addition to supplementing your child's brain development.

The schizophrenia study, like autism studies before it, found babies born to dark-skinned mothers are far more likely to develop the mental illness, and researchers believe this discovery of a sunlight factor could have huge implications for our society, as lead author McGrath notes:

"For example, in dark-skinned ethnic groups living in cold countries, there is a substantially increased risk of schizophrenia.[179] Kirkbride and Jones[180] have estimated

association of all-cause mortality with serum 25-hydroxyvitamin D in general practice, the CopD study," Durup et al, *Journal of Clinical Endocrinology & Metabolism*, August 2012, 97(8), doi: 10.1210jc.2012-1176

179   Black migrants are up to five times more likely to have schizophrenic children, "Schizophrenia and migration: a meta-analysis and review," Cantor-Graae E, Selten JP. *American Journal of Psychiatry*, 2005 Jan;162(1):12-24

180   "Foresight mental capital and wellbeing: discussion paper 12: putative prevention strategies to reduce serious mental illness in migrant and black and minority ethnic groups. London, England," Kirkbride JB, Jones PB.: Her Majesty's Stationary Office; 2008;

that if the yet-to-be-identified risk factors underlying the increased risk of schizophrenia in black minority ethnic groups living in England could be identified and prevented, it may be feasible to reduce the incidence of schizophrenia in this group by a staggering 87%.[181] While there is much more work to be done, if future studies confirm the association between developmental vitamin D deficiency and risk of schizophrenia, it raises the tantalizing prospect of the primary prevention of this disabling group of brain disorders in a manner comparable with folate supplementation and the prevention of spina bifida."

Apart from its work in the developing brain, vitamin D may confer protection in other ways, such as boosting immunity. Studies have shown that pregnant women who catch influenza are more at risk of having a schizophrenic child, therefore a vitamin that reduces your flu risk may also be reducing the risk of mental illness in your unborn child. The most important study to date on the topic reveals catching flu in the first trimester carries a 700% risk increase:

"The risk of schizophrenia was increased 7-fold for influenza exposure during the first trimester. There was no increased risk of schizophrenia with influenza

---

181   The "incidence" of schizophrenia is the rate of new diagnoses each year. The "prevalence" is the ratio of people living with the disorder at any given moment in time (total % of sufferers in the community)

during the second or third trimester. With the use of a broader gestational period of influenza exposure – early to midpregnancy – the risk of schizophrenia was increased 3-fold."[182]

Mothers should keep in mind, however, that the overall risk of schizophrenia is roughly one in a hundred. As we've already seen, the prevalence of autism is usually even higher, up to one in 60 in some countries, so there are very good reasons to ensure vitamin D intake is adequate.

After birth, there are also similar reasons to continue giving your children adequate vitamin D supplements:

"Vitamin D supplementation during the first year of life is associated with a reduced risk of schizophrenia in males. Preventing hypovitaminosis D [low vitamin D] during early life may reduce the incidence of schizophrenia."[183]

For parents wondering how to get vitamin D supplements into babies or children, the D3 capsules can simply be broken open and the powder mixed with food or milk according to taste.

So how much vitamin D is safe for a pregnant woman to take by supplement? The 400 or 500IU in most preg-

---

182   "Serologic evidence of prenatal influenza in the etiology of schizophrenia," Brown et al, *Archives of General Psychiatry*. 2004 Aug;61(8):774-80

183   "Vitamin D supplementation during the first year of life and risk of schizophrenia: a Finnish birth cohort study," McGrath et al, *Schizophrenia Research*, Volume 67, Issues 2–3, 1 April 2004, Pages 237–245

nancy multivitamins has virtually no effect in scientific trials. One randomised double-blind trial on vitamin D safety in pregnancy has just been completed. It tested hundreds of mothers on 400IU, 2000IU and 4000IU daily supplements, and found that 400IU failed to bring mothers up to the minimum recommended blood level of 80 nmol/L (32 ng/ml).

"Not a single adverse event was attributed to vitamin D supplementation or circulating 25(OH)D levels. It is concluded that vitamin D supplementation of 4000 IU/d for pregnant women is safe and most effective in achieving sufficiency in all women and their neonates regardless of race, whereas the current estimated average requirement (400IU) is comparatively ineffective at achieving adequate circulating 25(OH)D concentrations, especially in African Americans."[184]

The 4000IU dose succeeded in bringing women up to an average 50ng/ml (125 nmol/L) – about the equivalent of what adults should have with adequate sunlight exposure. Apart from minimising the risk of diseases like some of those listed above, good vitamin D levels in pregnancy appear to assist the placenta in priming baby's immune system.[185]

---

184   "Vitamin D supplementation during pregnancy: double-blind, randomized clinical trial of safety and effectiveness," Hollis et al, *Journal of Bone & Mineral Research*, 2011 Oct;26(10):2341-57. doi: 10.1002/jbmr.463
185   "Placenta-specific methylation of the vitamin D 24-hydroxylase gene: implications for feedback autoregulation of

Pregnant women with low vitamin D levels are up to four times more likely to end up having a caesarean section rather than a natural birth.[186] A low vitamin D reading is linked to pre-eclampsia and smaller than usual babies.[187]

Human trials on some aspects of vitamin D research are impossible, because of ethics considerations. For example, researchers can use pregnant mice and rats to experiment with – completely starving them of vitamin D on the one hand, or putting them under UV lamps for extended periods of time on the other – to test theories about how vitamin D works. They cannot carry out such controlled studies on pregnant women.

For that reason, when health officials demand more proof by way of "randomized, controlled human trials", sometimes they are asking for something that can never be done. The research in the nitty-gritty dangerous areas will only ever be observational, after the fact.

Nevertheless, what scientists are discovering in animal studies is that pregnant mice with low vitamin D have bad outcomes in their offspring:[188]

active vitamin D levels at the fetomaternal interface," Novakovic et al *J. Biol. Chem.* 2009, 284, 14838-14848

186   "Association between Vitamin D Deficiency and Primary Cesarean Section," Merewood et al, *The Journal of Clinical Endocrinology & Metabolism* March 1, 2009 vol. 94 no. 3 940-945

187   "Maternal vitamin D and fetal growth in early-onset severe preeclampsia," Robinson et al, presented at the 73rd Annual Meeting of the South Atlantic Association of Obstetricians and Gynecologists, Hot Springs, VA, Jan. 30-Feb. 2, 2011.

188   "The In Utero Effects of Maternal Vitamin D Deficiency

"This animal model is consistent with the fetal origins hypothesis, first articulated by David Barker, which postulates that in utero epigenetic fetal programming, as a result of environmental events during pregnancy, induces specific genes and genomic pathways that control fetal development and subsequent disease risk.[189] This hypothesis initially was applied to adult disorders, Type 2 diabetes mellitus, obesity, and heart disease, but is particularly applicable to asthma, since recurrent wheezing is prevalent in early life and most asthma is diagnosed by age 6 years. We believe that much, if not all, of the fetal origins hypothesis is mediated by vitamin D, as it has a known influence in all of the above named disorders."

Stripped of its medicalese, the implications are serious: what happens in the womb through a lack of vitamin D may affect a child for the rest of its life.

"The role of vitamin D during pregnancy and its effect on maternal and fetal health is just beginning to be understood," concludes Carol Wagner in her review. "In the last five years, there has been an explosion of published data concerning the immune effects of vitamin D, yet little is known in this regard about the specific

– How it Results in Asthma and Other Chronic Diseases," Weiss and Litonjua, American Journal Of Respiratory And Critical Care Medicine Vol 183 2011:1286-1287

189   "Fetal origins of adult disease: strength of effects and biological basis," Barker et al. *Int J Epidemiol* 2002; 31:1235–1239.

immune effects of vitamin D during pregnancy.

"What is clear, however, is that vitamin D deficiency during pregnancy is rampant throughout the world, including countries such as the United States and Great Britain. While there remains much to be discovered and learned about vitamin D's effect on the mother and her developing fetus, there is enough evidence to support the premise that deficiency is not healthful for either the mother or fetus."

An illustration of how much vitamin D plays a role in pregnancy and infancy hit news headlines in 2012:

"The season in which a baby is born apparently influences the risk of developing mental disorders later in life, suggests a large new study. The season of birth may affect everything from eyesight and eating habits to birth defects and personality later in life. Past research has also hinted the season one is born in might affect mental health."[190]

The source of that story is a study published April 2012, which examined the medical records of 29 million Brits, including a specific 58,000 strong cohort suffering from schizophrenia, bipolar disorder and recurrent depression. What they found is that all the main mental disorders can be pegged back to the season of birth.[191]

---

190   "Being born in winter can mess with your head," Charles Choi, *LivesScience.com*, 11 May 2012

191   "Seasonal Distribution of Psychiatric Births in England," Disanto et al, *PLoS ONE*, 7(4): e34866. doi:10.1371/journal.pone.0034866

Schizophrenia and bipolar, for example, are most often found in British residents born in January, at the peak of the northern winter, and least often found in people born in July, August and September, being the northern summer.

Depression peaks in May – the northern spring – with the fewest cases among people born in November. At first glance that seems to conflict with the vitamin D theory, but researchers say it's easily explained – developing fetal brains may need vitamin D at different times. Schizophrenia and bipolar patterns might be set in the first trimester which, for babies born in winter, occurs the previous spring when maternal vitamin D has hit rock bottom. Depression, on the other hand, might result from a lack of vitamin D in the second or third trimesters, which for May births coincides with winter.

"SC (Schizophrenia) births showed the most striking seasonality," reported the study. "These results are also consistent with those of a previous study of English SC patients born between 1921 and 1960 indicating that the season of birth effect is a stable feature of SC."

The odds of being born in winter for schizophrenia patients were 17% higher than being born in summer. Obviously people who go on to develop mental illness are being born year-round, but if most mothers are clinically deficient or insufficient in vitamin D all the time, then that's no great surprise. What the study shows is that the northern hemisphere summer gives enough of a vitamin D spike to some mothers to save their children from the increased risk.

Unfortunately a lack of vitamin D during pregnancy is like leaving the house unlocked. There's no guarantee a burglar is going to pick your house to raid on that particular day, but if he does he'll find it defenceless. That's what an increased risk is, it's not a certainty that fate [in the form of an environmental trigger] will strike you, but an increased possibility. With researchers now suggesting that vitamin D deficiency in the womb and early childhood could account for 44% of schizophrenia cases, the solution may be in the hands of mothers everywhere.

The British confirmation that mental illness is related to your birth season follows similar studies in the United States that made the same discovery.[192]

More tragically, researchers have found suicide follows the same pattern, with people born in April/May in the northern hemisphere more likely to end their own lives, and people born October/November less likely – very similar to the seasonal spread for Depression. [193]

To think that one vitamin, and whether you get enough of it in your mother's womb or not, can have such a huge impact on your life, is sobering to say the least.

192   "Birth seasonality in bipolar disorder, schizophrenia, schizoaffective disorder and stillbirths," Torrey et al, (1996). *Schizophr Res* 21: 141–149

193   "Effect of month of birth on the risk of suicide," Salib E, Cortina-Borja M (2006). *Br J Psychiatry* 188: 416–422

One area where vitamin D does not have an impact on otherwise-healthy kids is their academic ability. While the power of the vitamin to kickstart the brains of older people, and particularly Alzheimer's sufferers, is undeniable, new studies have shown it has no such effect on teenagers.

Whether that's because their bodies are being flooded with other hormones and influences isn't known. What we do know is that a British study found teens from more advantaged backgrounds had higher vitamin D3 levels (obtainable from sunlight or specific D3 supplements), whereas children from disadvantaged backgrounds tended to have the D2 variety, sourced from food.

When their high school exam results were assessed against their vitamin D levels, there was no difference between the groups.[194]

Keep taking the omega-3 pills, kids.

---

[194]   "Milk won't make kids Einsteins," *Daily RX News,* May 2012, www.dailyrx.com/news-article/vitamin-d-does-not-improve-academic-performance-or-brains-children-18580.html

Chapter 10

MENTAL ILLNESS

"Vitamin D deficiency and insufficiency are both highly prevalent in adolescents with severe mental illness"
— *BMC Journal of Psychiatry,* 2012

We've seen in the previous chapter how a lack of vitamin D during pregnancy can increase the risk of a child developing mental illness. The good news is that in some cases vitamin D can help bring mental illness under control.

The Endocrine Society conference in the US has heard how a group of three women previously diagnosed with major depressive disorder had their lives turned around by the sunshine vitamin. All were on anti-depressants, and had underlying medical conditions including Type 2 diabetes or an underactive thyroid.

Blood tests showed their vitamin D levels had dropped to between 8.9 ng/ml and 14.5 ng/ml – well into deficient and seriously deficient territory. After two to three months of vitamin D supplementation their serum 25(OH)D levels were restored to a healthy 32 to 38 ng/ml.

Using the Beck Depression Inventory, a 21-point survey that rates levels of depression and sadness, one patient moved from clinical severe depression (32 points at baseline) to mild depression (12 points) on completion. Another fell from 26 points (moderate depression) to 8 points (clinically minimal depression), while the third patient moved from moderate to mild.

Sonal Pathak, the US endocrinologist presenting the study, says the implications are fascinating and important:

"Vitamin D may have an as-yet-unproven effect on mood, and its deficiency may exacerbate depression… Screening at-risk depressed patients for vitamin D deficiency and treating it appropriately may be an easy and cost-effective adjunct to mainstream therapies for depression," he said.[195]

The impact of vitamin D deficiency is widespread. A New Zealand study has found the disorder is common in psychiatric inpatients, schizophrenics and in particular darker-skinned Maori patients.

---

195   "Treating vitamin D deficiency may improve depression among women," Allison Cerra, *DrugstoreNews,* www.drugstorenews. com/article/treating-vitamin-d-deficiency-may-improve-depression-among-women

The research, led by David Menkes at the Waikato Clinical School, reveals 91% of the 102 inpatients studied had sub-optimal (below 30 ng/ml) or deficient vitamin D. Broken down further, 74% were below 20 ng/ml (50 nmol/L), and 19% had less than 10 ng/ml (25 nmol/L).

Schizophrenics were most likely to be severely deficient – 34% of them fell into the lowest bracket compared with 9% of the rest. Bi-polar sufferers, whilst still deficient at 19.8 ng/ml, had the highest average vitamin D levels in the sample.

"The observed prevalence of vitamin D deficiency in our psychiatric inpatient population supports the idea that supplementation should be more generally available, and perhaps routinely prescribed, given its low cost, lack of adverse effects and multiple potential benefits," Menkes wrote in the study.[196]

An American study has reported similar results. Of 104 adolescents receiving acute mental health treatment, 34% had less than 20 ng/ml of vitamin D in their blood, 38% were sub-optimal (between 20 ng/ml and 30 ng/ml), with 28% normal.

Adolescents with psychotic behaviour were three and a half times more likely to be in the lowest vitamin D range.

---

196   "Vitamin D status of psychiatric inpatients in New Zealand's Waikato region," Menkes et al, *BMC Psychiatry*, June 2012, *BMC Psychiatry* 2012, 12:68 doi:10.1186/1471-244X-12-68 http://www.biomedcentral.com/content/pdf/1471-244X-12-68.pdf

"Vitamin D deficiency and insufficiency are both highly prevalent in adolescents with severe mental illness," they concluded.[197]

197   "Vitamin D and psychotic features in mentally-ill adolescents – a cross sectional study," Gracious et al, *BMC Psychiatry* 2012, 12:38

Chapter 11

MULTIPLE SCLEROSIS

"There is strong evidence that vitamin D concentrations during late adolescence and young adulthood have a major effect in determining MS risk"

– Lancet Neurology, 2010

For a long time, it's been known that the number of multiple sclerosis cases grows the further north or south of the equator you go. The disease, as it progresses, causes people increasing amounts of discomfort and pain as they undergo nerve damage. Sufferers live, on average, five to ten years less. In my experience it's worse than that: Fiona, a New Zealand TV colleague of mine, sister of a Hollywood movie director, passed away July 2012 after a long battle with MS – she'd been diagnosed in the early 1990s as I recall, when we were working together. She was only 50.

Fiona's story is not unique. She was one of millions of sufferers worldwide. Scotland has the highest per capita rate of the disease, with one in 500 people affected.

It's a neurological disease, resulting from the decay of myelin, a protective fatty sheath found around axons in the brain and spinal cord. Myelin helps nerves send messages across the body, so when it breaks down it's like the blue screen of death on a computer; your system slowly starts to malfunction, more and more often. In the early stages the discomfort can be mild tingling, but by the end it can be blindness, paralysis and death.

With a clear north-south spread, it didn't take long for researchers to pose the obvious question: is multiple sclerosis caused by a lack of vitamin D?[198]

For a start, the disease – like mental illness – can be tied back to the season of birth. Northern hemisphere sufferers are more likely to have been born around May, and least likely to have been born in November – the same season variation as that for depression.[199]

A 2006 study of US servicemen, based on routine blood samples taken and then comparing the results to later diagnoses, found a massive drop in multiple

---

198   The first scientific study to ask this question was in 1974: Goldberg P. Multiple sclerosis: vitamin D and calcium as environmental determinants of prevalence (a viewpoint). Part 1: sunlight, dietary factors and epidemiology. *Intern J Environ Stud* 1974; 6: 19–27.

199   "Timing of birth and risk of multiple sclerosis: population based study," Willer et al, *BMJ*. 2005 January 15; 330(7483): 120. doi: 10.1136/bmj.38301.686030.63

sclerosis cases the higher the vitamin D blood levels were.

Because of their jobs as active service personnel, the sample already had higher than average vitamin D levels. For example, the lowest 20% had vitamin D below 63.3 nmol/L (25.3 ng/ml), which is a much healthier bottom quintile than psychiatric patients enjoy, for example.

Nonetheless, the US study found service personnel with the highest levels, above 99 nmol/L (39.6 ng/L) reduced their risk of developing MS by 62%.[200]

Another study found children who played longer outside each day during summer, between the ages of 6 and 15, lowered their risk of developing multiple sclerosis by an incredible 69%. The researchers found it was even more important to ensure children got sun exposure in winter as well – another clue that vitamin D was a big player.[201]

Dermatologists and skin specialists might hate the idea, but the researchers independently discovered that

200   "Serum 25-Hydroxyvitamin D Levels and Risk of Multiple Sclerosis," Munger et al, *Journal of the American Medical Association, JAMA.* 2006;296(23):2832-2838. doi:10.1001/jama.296.23.2832

201   "Past exposure to sun, skin phenotype, and risk of multiple sclerosis: case-control study," van der Mei et al, *British Medical Journal*, 2003 August 9; 327(7410): 316. doi: 10.1136/bmj.327.7410.316, http://www.ncbi.nlm.nih.gov/pmc/articles/PMC169645/

people with higher skin damage from sunbathing were far less likely to contract multiple sclerosis than peaches and cream wallflowers – a 68% lower risk.

For children who develop multiple sclerosis, their vitamin D status has been shown to have a big impact on the intervals between relapses. For every 10 ng/ml that they increase their blood levels by, their risk of a relapse dropped by 34% in one American study.[202]

Mothers who drink more D-fortified milk during pregnancy have been shown to reduce the risk of multiple sclerosis in their children by 43%.[203]

All of the attention on vitamin D makes sense now, in the light of the latest major study to be released. Scientists at Oxford have found what they believe to be a "leading cause for multiple sclerosis", and it turns out to be a gene that causes vitamin D deficiency.[204]

"The study examined the DNA of a group of people with multiple sclerosis who also have a large number of family members with the disease," says Christina Galbraith, a spokeswoman for the Jeffrey Epstein VI

---

202   "Vitamin D status is associated with relapse rate in pediatric-onset multiple sclerosis," Mowry et al, *Annals of Neurology*, Volume 67, Issue 5, pages 618–624, May 2010

203   "Gestational vitamin D and the risk of multiple sclerosis in offspring," Mirzaei et al, *Annals of Neurology*, Volume 70, Issue 1, pages 30–40, July 2011

204   "A genetic cause for multiple sclerosis is identified and funded by science patron Jeffrey Epstein," news release, 16 June 2012, www.jeffreyepsteinfoundation.com

Foundation that part-funded the Oxford research with the Multiple Sclerosis Society.

"All the DNA samples showed a distortion of the CYP27B1 gene which controls vitamin D levels in the body.

"Despite this pivotal link, not all people with vitamin D deficiency develop multiple sclerosis…however, a distortion of the CYP27B1 gene is increasingly apparent in MS cases and it's possible that the gene generates other, yet undetected, complications that lead to the disease."

This, of course, reinforces the argument you've met repeatedly in this book, that whilst there may be environmental trigger points for various diseases – straws that break the camel's back – the camel is more vulnerable to those triggers because of a lack of vitamin D in the first place.

In the case of multiple sclerosis, it might be that some people develop it because of a simple lack of vitamin D and the introduction of a trigger, while others may develop it because their genes don't allow them to process vitamin D properly, thus also leaving them vulnerable when a trigger comes along. Treatment and prevention for each group might involve different strategies.

In the meantime, researchers say the evidence is almost overwhelming, and it's time for serious trials to get underway:

"Vitamin D supplementation in healthy individuals is emerging as a promising approach for MS prevention. In utero and early-life exposure could also be important, but *there is strong evidence that vitamin D concentrations during late adolescence and young adulthood have a major effect in determining MS risk.* [205]

"On the basis of the results of the only longitudinal study of serum 25-hydroxyvitamin D and MS onset,[206] and assuming that these results are unbiased and vitamin D is truly protective against MS, over 70% of MS cases in the USA and Europe could be prevented by increasing the serum 25-hydroxyvitamin D concentration of adolescents and young adults to above 100 nmol/L.[207] These concentrations are commonly found only in individuals with outdoor lifestyles in sunny regions, but could be reached in most people by taking 1000–4000 IU cholecalciferol daily.[208]

---

205 "Vitamin D and multiple sclerosis: a review," Ascherio et al, Lancet Neurol 2010; 9: 599–612, http://66.160.145.48/seaton/pdfs/27/Ascherio_2010.pdf

206 "Serum 25-hydroxyvitamin D levels and risk of multiple sclerosis," Munger et al. JAMA 2006; 296: 2832–38.

207 "Vitamin D deficiency: a worldwide problem with health consequences," Holick et al, Am J Clin Nutr 2008; 87 (suppl): 1080S–86S. See also "Vitamin D deficiency: a global perspective, Prentice A. Nutr Rev 2008; 66 (suppl 2): S153–64.

208 Hollis BW. Circulating 25-hydroxyvitamin D levels indicative of vitamin D sufficiency: implications for establishing a new effective dietary intake recommendation for vitamin D. J Nutr 2005; 135: 317–22.

"Whereas future observational epidemiological studies, and genetic and molecular investigations, will be useful to strengthen and refine the hypothesis, evidence is approaching equipoise,[209] at which the soundest decision might be to do a large randomised trial to establish the safety and efficacy needed to promote large-scale vitamin D supplementation.

"Although substantial evidence supports the safety of even large doses of vitamin D, such evidence is based on studies of limited size and duration, which were mostly done in older adults. A test of the hypothesis that vitamin D could reduce MS risk will require the administration of relatively high doses of vitamin D to hundreds of thousands of young adults for several years, and careful monitoring for unforeseen adverse effects is mandatory.

"Given the financial, logistical, and scientific complexity, and the limited societal experience with large-scale population experiments, we suggest that an international multi-disciplinary working group should be set up to oversee the design of future prevention or supplementation studies."

See also "Human serum 25-hydroxycholecalciferol response to extended oral dosing with cholecalciferol," Heaney et al, *Am J Clin Nutr* 2003; 77: 204–10.

209   The point at which medical researchers believe they have found the most successful treatment for a given condition and which they believe they are ethically-bound to make known and put into formal testing.

For researchers to state they are reaching "equipoise" on multiple sclerosis prevention is a major development, and not taken lightly. One of those human trials has just got underway in New Zealand and Australia – too late to save my colleague Fiona but not too late to save others.

This four year study, PrevANZ, is testing doses of vitamin D at three different levels – 1000IU daily, 5,000IU and 10,000IU, as well as placebo. Two hundred and ninety people who have experienced their first bout of the neurological precursor to MS, known as "clinically isolated syndrome", are taking part. Researchers will analyse the doses for safety over the four years, as well as whether they reduce relapses and reduce MS lesions that are visible in MRI scans.

The choice for readers is whether to wait four years to find out, or whether to now take a high dose of vitamin D daily after talking to your doctor, on the grounds of promoting great bone health, and on the offchance that the researchers are absolutely right about the protective effect of vitamin D.

Those most at risk of deficiency-related MS are teenagers and young adults.

Chapter 12

CHROHN'S DISEASE & TYPE 1 DIABETES

"Women with low vitamin D levels while pregnant have double the risk of giving birth to a diabetic child, when compared with mothers whose vitamin D levels were high"

– Diabetes, 2012

Yet another disease with a north-south gradient is Crohn's Disease, a debilitating autoimmune disorder of the bowel and gut that sees the body attack itself. Although people aged 15-35 are the most vulnerable, no one is safe and another age band it targets are fifty to seventy year olds.

Like MS, around one in 500 people are affected by it, and just like MS and virtually every other illness you've read about in this book, there's an inverse relationship between vitamin D status and risk of Crohn's or its other form, ulcerative colitis.

A study in the US found women aged 40+ with the highest levels of vitamin D in their blood (above 32 ng/ml or 80 nmol/L), reduced their chance of suffering Crohn's by 62%.[210]

It's long been known that people with Crohn's have particularly low vitamin D levels, so a couple of recent randomised controlled trials have tested vitamin D supplements on patients to see if they could stave off relapses.

A 2010 study gave 94 people either 1200IU of D3 a day or a placebo for a period of a year. All of them had Crohn's, and all were presently in a remission phase. The goal of the study was to find out which group lasted longest in remission.[211]

Twenty-nine percent of the placebo group relapsed within a year. Only 13 percent of the vitamin D3 group relapsed in that time, effectively a risk reduction of almost 70% – more than two thirds.

A smaller randomised study of fifteen Crohn's patients in the US who were not in remission, found high-dose vitamin D (10,000IU daily for 26 weeks) not only raised vitamin D levels substantially but it began pushing patients towards remission faster than those receiving only 1,000IU a day.[212]

---

210 "Higher Predicted Vitamin D Status Is Associated With Reduced Risk of Crohn's Disease," Ananthakrishna et al, *Gastroenterology*, Volume 142, Issue 3, March 2012, Pages 482–489
211 "Clinical trial: vitamin D3 treatment in Crohn's disease – a randomized double-blind placebo-controlled study," Jorgenson et al, *Alimentary Pharmacology & Therapeutics*, Volume 32, Issue 3, pages 377–383, August 2010
212 "Vitamin D may be easy, low-risk way to relieve symptoms

"This one nutritional supplementation actually made a real clinical impact without any toxicity," lead researcher Brian Bosworth told an American College of Gastroenterology meeting.

One of the ways that vitamin D is believed to work is anchored in its role as an immune system stimulant. It has the capability to force the human body to produce large amounts of natural antibiotics that can be used by the immune system and a type of white blood cell – macrophages – in their attacks on invading organisms.

"The net effect of these actions is to support increased bacterial killing in a variety of cell types. The efficacy of such a response is highly dependent on vitamin D status," reports researcher Martin Hewison in the journal *Nature*. "The potential importance of this mechanism as a determinant of human disease is underlined by increasing awareness of vitamin D insufficiency across the globe."[213]

The fact that Crohn's is an immunity disorder, that sufferers almost invariably have low levels of the vitamin, and that the vitamin is crucial to regulating our immune systems, gives what is called "biological plau-

---

of Crohn's disease," by Monica Smith, *Gastroenterology & Endoscopy News*, June 2012, Vol 63:6

213   "Antibacterial effects of vitamin D," Hewison, *Nature Reviews Endocrinology* 7, 337-345 (June 2011) | doi:10.1038/nrendo.2010.226

sibility" to the idea that 25(OH)D can impact Crohn's.

Clearly, it does. The 'why?' of it remains under investigation.

DIABETES

Another autoimmune disorder linked with low vitamin D is Type I Diabetes. This is the variant that often begins in childhood, what we used to call "sugar diabetes" because the body loses its ability to produce insulin, and children require daily injections.

Like Crohn's, MS and other similar disorders, Type I Diabetes likewise shows geographical and seasonal distribution patterns. Those clues now on the table, what have scientists learned?

For a start, there's clear evidence that giving your children regular vitamin D – either through sunlight or supplement or a combination of both, significantly reduces their risk of becoming diabetic. One study published in the Lancet found parents who regularly gave their kids 2000IU of vitamin D cut the prospect of Type I Diabetes by 78%.[214]

In another meta-analysis study, which did not break down dosages, children supplemented with vitamin D of any kind and amount reduced their risk of diabetes by 29%.[215]

---

214   "Intake of vitamin D and risk of type 1 diabetes: a birth-cohort study," Hypponen et al, *Lancet* 2001;358:1500-3.
215   "Vitamin D supplementation in early childhood and risk

The protective effect should, ideally, begin in pregnancy. A just-published study reveals women with low vitamin D levels while pregnant have double the risk of giving birth to a diabetic child, when compared with mothers whose vitamin D levels were high.[216]

"Type 1 diabetes is an autoimmune disease that is one of the most common chronic diseases during childhood. With the exception of certain susceptibility genes, the causes of type 1 diabetes are essentially unknown," reported the study.

It's the first study in the world to directly link a lack of vitamin D during pregnancy to a significant risk of Type I Diabetes, and flies in the face of some earlier research, but the study authors say their process was more thorough:

"These previous studies are not directly comparable with ours, because we have not only measured maternal 25-OH D but also followed the children until they were 15 years of age, with respect to the onset of clinical type 1 diabetes."

And the size of their study was formidable. Blood samples taken from more than 30,000 Norwegian

of type 1 diabetes: a systematic review and meta-analysis," C S Zipitis & A K Akobeng, *Arch Dis Child* 2008;93:512-517 doi:10.1136/adc.2007.128579

216   "Maternal Serum Levels of 25-Hydroxy-Vitamin D During Pregnancy and Risk of Type 1 Diabetes in the Offspring," Sorenson et al, *Diabetes*, January 2012 vol. 61 no. 1 175-178, http://diabetes.diabetesjournals.org/content/61/1/175.full

mothers twenty years ago and stored, were reanalysed and matched against outcomes from those babies. Being a notifiable disease in Norway, it was easy for researchers to identify virtually every child who had developed diabetes by the age of 15, and track them back to their mothers' blood samples.

Chapter 13

SUNSCREENS:
A CLEAR AND PRESENT DANGER

"Using sunscreen has not been shown to prevent melanoma or basal cell carcinoma"

– American Academy of Pediatricians, 2011

It seems such an easy message to sell: Slip, slop, slap. The idea of using a chemical lotion to block harmful UV rays as a primary method of sun protection has a lot of simple appeal. Clearly, people using sunscreen don't burn and they can easily spot the convenience and health benefits of that particular outcome. To that extent, sunscreen sells itself as users become reliant on it to help maintain an outdoor lifestyle for themselves and their families. But here's the rub: there's strong scientific evidence that sunscreens don't actually work against the most dangerous skin cancers, and there's strong emerging evidence that sunscreens may actually contain toxic particles that cause cancer and other genetic damage.

First, however, a little history.

In 1935, your chance of developing melanoma in your lifetime was around 1:1500. Today, melanoma risk has ballooned to 1:33 for a baby born now.[217] Why such a huge rise in risk?

The first commercial sunscreen was invented in 1938 by chemistry student Franz Greiter, who allegedly received a sunburn while climbing Piz Buin in the Swiss Alps that inspired him to develop a protective lotion.

Also from the necessity-is-the-mother-of-invention file, US WWII serviceman Benjamin Green – apparently sick of getting sunburnt while fighting in the Pacific – developed his own sunscreen independently in 1944 based on red petroleum jelly, which later became the stepping stone for Coppertone to develop its range of sunscreens.

You won't find the ingredients used in those first sunscreens in any products available today. Para-aminobenzoic acid, or PABA, for example, was patented in 1943 and whilst being a good UVB barrier, often used in sunscreens and women's cosmetics, it has subsequently been found to degrade when exposed to sunlight and may be carcinogenic under certain circumstances[218],

---

217   "Cutaneous ultraviolet exposure and its relationship to the development of skin cancer", Rigel DS, *J Am Acad Dermatol.* 2008: 58(5 suppl 2):S129-S132) http://www.sciencedirect.com/science/article/pii/S0190962207024139

218   A 2005 study found PABA caused thyroid cancer in rats, "Promotion of thyroid carcinogenesis by para-aminobenzoic acid in

which somewhat defeats the purpose. It is banned in Europe, and no longer used in many other regions.

Sunscreens have gone through a multitude of formulations in the attempt for the perfect lotion, but so far no one has cracked it. There are two varieties available to consumers, organic-based lotions or mineral based. The organically-derived sunscreens rely on the following FDA-approved[219] chemical compounds:

Cinoxate

Ensulizole

Homosalate

Octinoxate

Octocrylene

Padimate O

Para-aminobenzoic acid (PABA)

Trolamine

Those compounds just listed are only effective against UVB radiation. They will not block any UVA radiation at all.

There are a further subset of organic molecules that sunscreen manufacturers have found have some limited effect on UVA rays:

Dioxybenzone

---

rats initiated with N-bis(2-hydroxypropyl)nitrosamine", Hasumara et al, *Toxicological Sciences*, 2005 Jul;86(1):61-7. Epub 2005 Apr 20

219   Other countries, like the UK, Europe, New Zealand and Australia, in some cases permit other compounds to be used in sunscreens that are not approved for human use in the USA.

Oxybenzone

Sulibenzone

Those chemicals are effective against UVB and UVA-2 radiation frequencies, but not effective against UVA-1 frequencies. L'Oreal has developed a couple of chemicals that are only effective against UVA-2 radiation (again, to a limited extent), but there is only one organic compound approved in the US that is effective in any way against UVA-1 radiation: Avobenzone.[220]

The problem with many of these organic (mostly benzene-based) sunscreen compounds is that they are prone to "photodegradation", or breaking down when exposed to sunlight.

"Controversy," reports one recent scientific study, "has also developed regarding the possibility of adverse biological effects from various ingredients in sunscreens. Oxybenzone, an ingredient widely used in sunscreens, is purported to have a potentially disruptive effect on hormonal homeostasis."

What scientists have found is that Oxybenzone (aka Benzophenone-3) is well and truly absorbed into the human body through the skin, after being applied in sunscreens. It has turned up in the urine and blood of 96.8% of people tested, and is believed to accumulate in vital organs like the kidney, liver, spleen and male testes, but also in the intestines, stomach, heart and adrenal glands. It has been linked in one scientific

220   Also known on labels as Butyl Methoxydibenzoylmethane

study to low birth weight in babies.[221]

What does it do? We know it has an estrogen like effect and has been scientifically shown to stimulate human breast cancer cells[222] – not necessarily a good thing if you are at risk of developing breast cancer, as many women are. It also gives men an extra tweak of estrogen and displays – at a biochemical level – what scientists call "anti androgenic" or feminising hormonal effects.

A study of 15 young males and 17 post-menopausal females over two weeks measured statistically signifi-cant hormonal changes after using oxybenzone, but not enough to cause what scientists call "clinically significant perturbations". In other words, while the sunscreen chemical is affecting our bodies, this tiny study of 32 people didn't detect anything requiring treatment or intervention. What of the effect on babies or children, however? We don't know. We do know that sunscreen ingredients are now being found in human breast milk.[223]

---

221   http://www.ewg.org/analysis/toxicsunscreen
222   "Metabolism of 2-hydroxy-4-methoxybenzophenone in isolated rat hepatocytes and xenoestrogenic effects of its metabolites on MCF-7 human breast cancer cells", Nakagawa & Suzuki, *Chem Biol Interactions Journal*, 2002; 139:115-128. See also "UV filters with antagonistic action at androgen receptors etc", Ma et al, *Toxicological Sciences*, 2003; 74:43-50. See also "Additive estrogenic effects of mixtures of frequently used UV filters on pS2-gene transcription in MCF-7 cells," Heneweer et al, *Toxicol Appl Pharmacol* 2005; 208:170-177
223   American Academy of Pediatrics, http://aapnews.

One scientific study on human wastewater outflows into rivers has found however that all that oxybenzone we are absorbing and excreting is having a horrific effect on marine life, dramatically reducing the fertility of trout and other fish species exposed to oxybenzone.[224]

In the interests of balance, a further analysis has worked out it could take up to 277 years for a woman using sunscreen every day to finally get enough of a build-up of oxybenzone to harm her, pointing out that what is toxic to small animals is not necessarily so to humans.[225]

What we do know, however, is that oxybenzone may become ineffective and even toxic under normal sunscreen use conditions. A just-released study has tested what happens to oxybenzone sunscreens when their users jump into chlorinated swimming pools or spas. The chlorine reacted with the oxybenzone and "caused significantly more cell death than unchlorinated controls…Exposing a commercially available sunscreen product to chlorine also resulted in decreased UV absorbance, loss of UV protection, and

aappublications.org/content/32/3/32.short

224   "Estrogenic activity and reproductive effects of the UV-filter oxybenzone (2-hydroxy-4-methoxyphenyl-methanone) in fish", Coronado et al, *Aquatic Toxicology*, Volume 90, Issue 3, 21 November 2008, Pages 182–187

225   "Safety of Oxybenzone: Putting Numbers Into Perspective", Wang et al, *Archives of Dermatology*, 2011;147(7):865-866. doi:10.1001/archdermatol.2011.173

enhanced cytotoxicity [meaning it becomes poisonous to human cells]."[226]

There are question marks about the safety of other ingredients in organic sunscreens.

"Retinyl palmitate, a compound used extensively in various cosmetic and personal care products, has received wide attention as a potential photocarcinogen (light-activated carcinogen)."

This chemical has been shown to have carcinogenic properties in animal testing, and it also has been shown to create harmful free radicals[227] in the skin as a result of breaking down under UV exposure. Scientific reaction is mixed however, with some suggesting that other antioxidant compounds in the human skin should be

---

226   "Altered UV absorbance and cytotoxicity of chlorinated sunscreen agents", Sherwood et al, *Journal of Cutaneous and Ocular Toxicology*, 2012, January 18, http://www.ncbi.nlm.nih.gov/pubmed/22257218

227   Free radicals are loose electrons within an atom or molecular structure that makes the structure "reactive" until it finds equilibrium, usually by breaking another nearby chemical bond to restore its positive or negative charge to neutral. These things are all well and good until the structure they react with is a cell within your body, because the resulting damage can cause cancer or interfere with other body functions. We use antioxidants to try and mop up these free radicals by providing them with something to bind with that isn't part of you, but it's hit and miss. There is no guarantee that free radicals created by UV breaking down sunscreen, will necessarily bind with antioxidants – like a lightning bolt in search of the quickest route to the ground, a free radical will break whatever is easiest and closest at the relevant moment.

capable of protecting against damage caused by retinyl palmitate generated free radicals,[228] and they also argue that the mice in the cancer tests were prone to skin cancer anyway.

Like oxybenzone, in the absence of seriously hard evidence showing the compound is definitely harmful, retinyl palmitate will remain in sunscreens used by adults and children.

In 2005 a series of experiments using sunscreen containing octocrylene, octylmethoxycinnamate and benzophenone-3 revealed that within one hour of application according to manufacturer's instructions, the chemicals were generating more "reactive oxygen species"(ROS) in the skin than people wearing no sunscreen were getting via direct UV radiation. In other words, the sunscreen was acting like oil in a frypan in terms of its effect on users' skin and resultant ROS damage.[229] It's one of the reasons health authorities now seek regular re-application of yet more chemicals every hour or so, locking sunscreen users into a vicious circle.

The second category of sun screens, the mineral-based ones, have issues of their own. These are the Zinc Oxide and Titanium Dioxide sun blocks. Unlike

228   "Current sunscreen controversies: a critical review", Burnett & Wang, *Photodermatology, Photoimmunology & Photomedicine,* 2011; 27: 58-67

229   "Sunscreen enhancement of UV-induced reactive oxygen species in the skin", Hanson et al, *Free Radical Biology and Medicine,* Volume 41, Issue 8, 15 October 2006, Pages 1205–1212

the organics, the Zinc and Titanium formulations were not thought to break down in sunlight and cause damage on the skin, meaning they stay protective for longer. However, in the race to become more effective these sunscreens deliver their active ingredients as nanoparticles – molecular compounds so small they can potentially pass through barriers like the human skin. Researchers have shown that when Titanium dioxide is stimulated by UV rays, its electrons become more energised and can "react with nearby oxygen and hydrogen compounds to produce highly reactive free radical compounds...when in contact with our skin these radicals can oxidise and reduce compounds including DNA, resulting in significant mutagenesis [causes mutations at a cellular level]."[230] Additionally, the resulting free radicals can react with organic sunscreen ingredients to create acids.

All of this is happening on and possibly under your skin unseen, of course, whilst you and your children happily sunbathe or play on the beach.

More than one research team has pointed out that the race to nanotechnology in sunscreens and cosmetics has been done "with no regard to the potential health risks."[231]

"Much concern has been voiced that the integration of nano-material technology into everyday formula-

---

230   "Sunscreen – a catch 22", Blum & Larsen, *Young Scientists Journal*, 2010, issue 8:11-14
231   Ibid

tions has outpaced the body of research evaluating their safety," echo Burnett & Wang, who nonetheless reach the conclusion that sunscreens should still be used regardless.[232]

Sadly, health agencies in Europe, Japan, Australia and New Zealand have been so keen to promote sunscreens that they have allowed products to go to market untested in regard to whether their ingredients may in fact cause cancer in their own right. Even in the US most ingredients have not been required to pass official safety tests.

Scientists now know that Zinc Oxide does in fact break down under UVB light, shedding zinc (Zn^{2+}). One study found "a reduction in cell viability" as a result and that Zinc oxide breakdown "causes cytotoxicity and oxidative stress [the generation of free radicals]."[233]

Another recent study paints an even more disturbing picture – actual genetic damage resulting from nano-technology in sunscreens and makeup. Remember, it is DNA damage that leads to skin cancer and melanoma, so this is where speculation about sunscreens possibly causing skin cancer is focused.

"Due to the extremely small size of the nanoparticles

232   "Current sunscreen controversies: a critical review", Burnett & Wang, *Photodermatology, Photoimmunology & Photomedicine*, 2011; 27: 58-67

233   "UV irradiation-induced zinc dissociation from commercial zinc oxide sunscreen etc", Martorano et al, *Journal of Cosmetic Dermatology*, vol 9, issue 4, Dec 2010:276-286

(NPs) being used, there is a concern that they may interact directly with macromolecules such as DNA," notes the study, published in the journal *Toxicology Letters.*[234]

"The present study was aimed to assess the genotoxicity of zincoxide (ZnO) NPs, one of the widely used ingredients of cosmetics, and other dermatological preparations in human epidermal cell line (A431). A reduction in cell viability as a function of both NP concentration as well as exposure time was observed."

The findings warn that Zinc oxide nanoparticles, "even at low concentrations, possess a genotoxic potential" capable of genetically mutating or harming human skin. "Hence, caution should be taken in their use in dermatological preparations as well as while handling."

This again raises valid questions about whether sunscreens are safe to use on infants and children, let alone adults.

"Although toxicity in infants or young children resulting from sunscreen absorption has not been reported," writes Dr Sophie Balk, "skin permeability to topically applied products is of concern in the very young, especially in preterm infants. Absorptive and other properties of children's skin may differ from those of adult skin

---

234   "DNA damaging potential of zincoxide nanoparticles in human epidermal cells," Sharma et al, *Toxicology Letters*, Volume 185, Issue 3, 28 March 2009, Pages 211–218

until children are at least 2 years old."[235]

Thomas Faunce, a biomedicine legal expert based at Australian National University in Canberra, says authorities may need to step up.

"It may be time for Australian safety regulators to apply the precautionary principle in this contact and increase labelling requirements about the use of nanoparticles in sunscreens."[236]

The problem is, how do you tackle the problem when health authorities, manufacturers and cancer charities are all financially in bed with each other?

Australia and New Zealand's cancer societies, for example, earn millions of dollars a year marketing their own range of sunscreen products. One of those, like similar products in the US and elsewhere, is a combination SPF30+ sunscreen and insect repellent. It contains the insecticide "Deet", known to science as diethyl toluamide, and the sunscreen octyl-methoxy-cinnamate. Ignore the fact that these two chemicals or their derivatives, when mixed together, can be poten-tially harmful.[237] Instead, note that the combo also lists

235   "Ultraviolet radiation reports shine light on how pediatricians can help patients avoid skin cancer," Sophie Balk MD, American Academy of Pediatrics, 2011

236   "Exploring the safety of nanoparticles in Australian sunscreens", Faunce, *International Journal of Biomedical Nanoscience and Nanotechnology*, Vol 1, no. 1, 2010:87-94, doi 10.1504/IJBNN.2010.034127

237   "Evaluation of percutaneous absorption of the repellent diethyltoluamide and the sunscreen ethylhexyl

an ingredient called piperonyl butoxide,[238] otherwise known as PBO, which is often added to "natural" insect sprays.

A 2011 study – the first of its kind – found this supposedly environmentally friendly chemical PBO appears to be as toxic to infants and children as letting them lick lead paint. The study found a four point drop in mental development levels for children whose homes are exposed to piperonyl butoxide in insect spray dispensers.[239]

Whilst that particular study was looking at the toxicity of PBO inhaled from automatic household spray dispensers, the application of the product directly on the skin in a sunscreen could also possibly leach it into the bloodstream, particularly of pregnant women or children. You are also likely to find PBO in headlice treatments for children.

"Children who were more highly exposed to PBO in personal air samples (≥4.34 ng/m3) scored 3.9 points lower on the Mental Developmental Index than those with lower exposures.[240]

p-methoxycinnamate-loaded solid lipid nanoparticles: an in-vitro study," Puglia et al, *J Pharm Pharmacol*. 2009 Aug;61(8):1013-9

238   See ingredient list, Cancer Council of Australia supplier, http://www.skinhealth.com.au/site/repelplus.html

239   "Impact of prenatal exposure to piperonyl butoxide and permethrin on 36-month neurodevelopment", Horton et al, *Pediatrics*. 2011 Mar;127(3):e699-706 http://www.ncbi.nlm.nih.gov/pubmed/21300677

240   "Natural insect sprays may be as toxic to children as lead paint – Study", *InvestigateDaily*, 14 Dec 2011, http://www.

"This drop in IQ points is similar to that observed in response to lead exposure," lead researcher Megan Horton of Columbia's Mailman School of Public Health told journalists. "While perhaps not impacting an individual's overall function, it is educationally meaningful and could shift the distribution of children in the society who would be in need of early intervention services".[241]

You might be surprised to discover that – despite being approved for use in households and on children – no significant human safety testing of PBO has ever taken place until the 2011 study.[242] And that's kind of the main point here – pesticide and sunscreen manufacturers have been given free rein to use the public as guinea pigs.

The New Zealand Cancer Society helpfully publishes a "materials safety sheet" on the ingredients of its products. The poisons information in the sheet

---

investigatemagazine.co.nz/Investigate/?p=2078

241   A study published May 2012 has followed the *Pediatrics* results up, and found PBO damages "critical neurological development", see "The Insecticide Synergist Piperonyl Butoxide Inhibits Hedgehog Signaling: Assessing Chemical Risks," Wang et al, *Toxicological Sciences, (2012) doi: 10.1093/toxsci/kfs165* http://toxsci.oxfordjournals.org/content/early/2012/05/03/toxsci.kfs165.short

242   On the other hand, scientists now know that piperonyl butoxide is also "immunotoxic" to fish, see "Immunotoxic and cytotoxic effects of atrazine, permethrin and piperonylbutoxide to rainbow trout following in vitro exposure," Shelley et al, *Fish & Shellfish Immunology*, Volume 33, Issue 2, August 2012, Pages 455–458

states the combined sunscreen and insect repellent is "not suitable for babies and toddlers". Great advice, and it was delivered to the Cancer Society in October 2009,[243] but it does not appear anywhere as a warning on the tube of sunscreen on sale in 2012. Thousands of families are likely to have used this harmful product on and around their children. Indeed, the tube labelling in NZ states "use this sunscreen in conjunction with other sunsmart behaviour", including "keep infants in the shade", clearly implying to me that it is safe for children as part of a mix of precautions.

The Cancer Council of Australia's PBO-containing product describes itself as "Ideal for families and child-care centers" in a description for the 500ml pump-bottle version.[244]

The Cancer Council defends its use of nanoparticles on its website:[245]

"Nanotechnology has been used in sunscreens for many years. To date, our assessment, drawing on the best available evidence, is that nanoparticulates used in sunscreens do not pose a risk. However, we continue

---

243   Based on the creation and modification dates of the PDF on the Cancer Society website, accessed June 2012. See http://www.cancernz.org.nz/assets/files/products/Insect_Repellent-MSDS-091013.pdf

244   See Cancer Council of Australia supplier, http://www.skinhealth.com.au/site/repelplus.html

245   http://www.cancer.org.au/cancersmartlifestyle/SunSmart/nanoparticles_sunscreen.htm

to monitor research and welcome any new research that sheds more light on this topic.

"Sunscreen formulas and their components are regulated through the Therapeutic Goods Administration (TGA). In early 2009, the TGA conducted an updated review of the scientific literature in relation to the use of nanoparticulate zinc oxide and titanium dioxide in sunscreens.

"The TGA review concluded that:

- The potential for titanium dioxide and zinc oxide nanoparticles in sunscreens to cause adverse effects depends primarily upon the ability of the nanoparticles to reach viable skin cells; and
- To date, the current weight of evidence suggests that titanium dioxide and zinc oxide nanoparticles do not reach viable skin cells; rather, they remain on the surface of the skin and in the outer layer of the skin that is composed of non-viable cells."

That review was conducted in early 2009. Evidently nothing further has been done by Australasian authorities. Yet in late 2009 this study was released:[246]

Titanium dioxide (TiO_2) nanoparticles, found in everything from cosmetics to sunscreen to paint to

---

246 "Nanoparticles Used in Common Household Items Cause Genetic Damage in Mice," ScienceDaily Nov. 17, 2009

vitamins, caused systemic genetic damage in mice, according to a comprehensive study conducted by researchers at UCLA's Jonsson Comprehensive Cancer Center.

"The TiO2 nanoparticles induced single- and double-strand DNA breaks and also caused chromosomal damage as well as inflammation, all of which increase the risk for cancer. The UCLA study is the first to show that the nanoparticles had such an effect, said Robert Schiestl, a professor of pathology, radiation oncology and environmental health sciences, a Jonsson Cancer Center scientist and the study's senior author.

Once in the system, the TiO2 nanoparticles accumulate in different organs because the body has no way to eliminate them. And because they are so small, they can go everywhere in the body, even through cells, and may interfere with subcellular mechanisms.

The study appeared the week of November 16 in the journal Cancer Research.

In the past, these TiO2 nanoparticles have been considered non-toxic in that they do not incite a chemical reaction. Instead, it is surface interactions that the nanoparticles have within their environment- in this case inside a mouse—that is causing the genetic damage, Schiestl said. They wander throughout the body causing oxidative stress, which can lead to cell death.

It is a novel mechanism of toxicity, a physico-chemical reaction, these particles cause in comparison to regular chemical toxins, which are the usual subjects of toxicological research, Schiestl said.

"The novel principle is that titanium by itself is chemically inert. However, when the particles become progressively smaller, their surface, in turn, becomes progressively bigger and in the interaction of this surface with the environment oxidative stress is induced," he said. "This is the first comprehensive study of titanium dioxide nanoparticle-induced genotoxicity, possibly caused by a secondary mechanism associated with inflammation and/or oxidative stress. Given the growing use of these nanoparticles, these findings raise concern about potential health hazards associated with exposure."

How do we reconcile studies like that with marketing campaigns telling parents to use titanium dioxide sunscreens on their children? It is true that studies so far have not found penetration of zinc or titanium through the skin barrier beyond 17 layers, but those tests have been done on adult skin, not infant skin, which is much less developed. Additionally, young children and particularly babies may suck skin with sunblock on, therefore ingesting the chemicals. Given that titanium dioxide nanoparticles are also used as a whitener in toothpaste, perhaps there's a different avenue for concern, although that's another story!

What it all comes back to, in the end, is that warning that nanotechnology usage has exploded into the community long before safety has been definitively proven. If sunscreens were a dead cert, 100% effective barrier to melanoma and all other skin cancers, you might look at the odds and say it's worth using them. Sunscreens don't prevent most skin cancers, however, and on current evidence might (either directly or indirectly) cause rather than prevent melanoma, so the risk/benefit ratio might be harder for parents to assess.

That's not the only concern, however.

Virtually every one of the NZ Cancer Society sunscreens (and a number of the Australian ones) also contains Vitamin E as an antioxidant, but there are no warnings on the packs[247] about the possible dangers of Vitamin E to men at risk of prostate cancer. A recent study found men using Vitamin E suffered a significant 17% increase in risk of developing prostate cancer, meaning you would not want to be using it daily in a sunscreen as recommended by health authorities. As the study warns: "Dietary supplementation with

---

247   As displayed in the ingredients lists on the NZ Cancer Society website, http://www.cancernz.org.nz/products/technical-info/ as retrieved in June 2012

vitamin E significantly increased the risk of prostate cancer among healthy men." [248]

Prostate cancer rates have – like melanoma – gone through the roof in the past three decades. Are sunscreens partly to blame? *The Journal of Cosmetic Dermatology* has previously reported that Vitamin E is absorbed into the human body at a level eleven times greater when applied to the skin, as compared to taking it in dietary supplement form. [249]

This is not to pick on the Australia or New Zealand cancer societies, by the way. The formulations in their products are similar to those used by other commercial suppliers. Don't assume that just because a product is marketed by reputable companies or charities, advertised on TV and sold in supermarkets that it is actually 100% risk-free. Do your homework.

Then there's the strange case of gardeners and agriculturalists, many of whom use herbicides or pesticides of some kind as part of their work. A 2004 study revealed sunscreens act like an open door for poisonous chemicals to penetrate your skin. The herbicide in question was 2,4-D – which forms one half of the deadly

---

248   "Vitamin E and the Risk of Prostate Cancer", Klein et al, *Journal of the American Medical Assn* (JAMA), October 12, 2011, Vol 306, No. 14, http://jama.jamanetwork.com/article.aspx?articleid=1104493

249   "Photodamage of the skin: protection and reversal with topical antioxidants", Burke, K E. *J Cosmet Dermatol.* 2004 Jul;3(3):149-55

"Agent Orange" formula. There was a 60% increase in the amount of herbicide that penetrated the skin via sunscreen, compared with no sunscreen, resulting in what researchers called "penetration enhancement" that showed "physical damage" to the skin.[250]

As you can see then, there are nagging concerns about whether sunscreens might actually be toxic, and whether they open gateways for other toxins. What comes next, however, is a bigger problem for the sunscreen industry: do they actually work? What you are about to read may astound you.

---

250   "Active ingredients in sunscreens act as topical penetration enhancers for the herbicide 2,4-dichlorophenoxyacetic acid", Pont et al, *Toxicology & Applied Pharmacology.* 2004 Mar 15;195(3):348-54

Chapter 14

MELANOMA: COULD SUNSCREENS BE CAUSING IT?

"The factor most significantly associated with increased melanoma risk was the use of sunscreens. Subjects who often used sunscreens had an increased odds ratio of 3.47 (three and a half times more risk) compared with subjects who never used sunscreens"

– Journal of Melanoma Research, 1998

The best explanation for why melanoma rates have skyrocketed since 1935 may be a relatively simple one: there's no hard evidence that sunscreens protect you against melanoma.

Think about that for a moment, let it sink in.

Numerous scientific studies have failed to find evidence that sunscreens are effective against the risk of developing the deadliest skin cancer, melanoma. In fact, in some cases, they have found sunscreen users have a significantly higher risk of developing melanoma.

A telltale sign of growing risk are what are called "nevi" – the brownish skin lesions like moles or dark freckles that can often morph into melanoma. A Canadian study of school children using SPF-30 broad spectrum sunscreen in randomised, controlled conditions over a three year period found regular sunscreen users did have "a slight decrease" in the number of new nevi on their skin, "however, this effect was seen only in children with freckles". In other words, for everyone else, sunscreen use failed to prevent the development of melanoma precursors.[251]

"In a large European study of white school-age children," report Jou et al in their June 2012 study, "sunscreen use was associated with an increased number of nevi."

In 2000, the *International Journal of Cancer* reported similar findings after a study involving nearly 1,500 people in Sweden.

"Persons who used sunscreens did not have a decreased risk of malignant melanoma. Instead, a significantly elevated odds-ratio (nearly double) for developing malignant melanoma after regular sunscreen use was found."[252]

---

251 "UV protection and sunscreens: What to tell patients", Jou et al, *Cleveland Clinic Journal of Medicine*, Vol 79, number 6, June 2012, pp427-436

252 "Sunscreen use and malignant melanoma", Westerdahl et al, *International Journal of Cancer*, 1 July 2000, Vol 87, issue 1, pp145-150

Even more disturbing for readers, the massive increase in melanoma risk for sunscreen users took place even though participants "did not suffer from sunburns while using sunscreens".

The only good news from scientific studies of sunscreen effectiveness is that the lotions are effective at helping prevent one of the main skin cancers, known as squamous cell carcinomas. These are very slow-growing cancers which, whilst they can spread, usually don't before they are diagnosed. Sunscreens don't protect you from the most common skin cancer – basal cell carcinoma – or the most deadly, melanoma. Sunscreens should carry warning labels to this effect, like cigarette packets, but they don't.

This refusal by manufacturers and health authorities to spell out the ineffectiveness is all the more inexplicable when you consider that every summer it is the sad and tragic stories of youthful melanoma victims that are trotted out to the news media and the public as the figureheads of sun safety messages urging people to buy and use sunscreen.

These latest studies have prompted the American Academy of Pediatricians to announce recently: "Correctly using sunscreen can prevent sunburn and is believed to protect against SCC. Using sunscreen has not, however, been shown to prevent melanoma or basal cell carcinoma."[253]

---

253   "Ultraviolet radiation reports shine light on how pediatricians

Remember, it is primarily melanoma that kills. The sunscreen in your cupboard is not lowering your risk of dying from skin cancer, no matter how many times a smiling person on TV urges you to slop on the sunscreen because of the dangers of melanoma. At best, the protective effects of sunscreen appear to be largely cosmetic in terms of slowing down solar aging. But at worst, sunscreens may be dangerously lulling you into complacency. Could it be that our massive melanoma rates are largely the result of a worldwide public health campaign encouraging people to use sunscreens that turn out to have been ineffective against melanoma?

Even the effectiveness against SCC cancers is far from total. A reduction of only 40% amongst people who use sunscreen religiously and well, still leaves a substantial relative risk of developing it.

It's not the first time a major public health awareness campaign has been launched on the back of erroneous data and backfired tragically. Another live example that many readers will be familiar with is the global promotion of condoms in "safe sex" campaigns. Medical studies actually show condoms are next to useless against many sexually transmitted infections, with the result that sexual infection statistics have risen rapidly amongst teenagers who've been lulled into a false sense of security because of desires by health authorities to

can help patients avoid skin cancer", Sophie J. Balk, M.D., FAAP, http://aapnews.aappublications.org/content/32/3/32.short

present simple, dumbed-down safe sex messages.[254]

In the case of melanoma, the embarrassment for public health officials actually gets even worse. Studies are showing that – ironically – people who get the most exposure to the sun are more likely to survive melanoma if they develop it, than people who slip, slop, slap religiously.

Let that one sink in for a moment as well.

If you regularly sunbathe and build up a tan and vitamin D reserves, your chances of surviving melanoma are much higher than if you are a 50 year old wallflower with the skin of a 20 year old who has sheltered away from the sun all her life. Researchers at the University of Leeds discovered this in a major study published in conjunction with the US National Institutes of Health in September 2009. People who regularly sunbathed and got melanoma were found 30% more likely to survive than non-sunbathers.[255]

Part of the reason for this enigma appears to be, yet again, the protective effect of vitamin D. Melanoma patients found to have the highest levels of vitamin D in their blood turned out to have the thinnest mela-

---

254   "Where the Rubba Meets The Road", Wishart & Morrow, *Investigate* magazine, July 2005, http://issuu.com/iwishart/docs/ investigate_july05/39

255   "Serum 25-Hydroxyvitamin D3 Levels are Associated With Breslow Thickness At Presentation and Survival From Melanoma", Newton-Bishop et al, *Journal of Clinical Oncology*, 21 September 2009, DOI:10.1200/JCO.2009.22.1135

noma lesions on their skin – and the shallower the melanoma the less risk there is of it spreading deeper and further into the body.

"Higher [vitamin D3] levels, at diagnosis, are associated with both thinner tumours and better survival from melanoma," reported the Leeds study. "Patients with melanoma, and those at high risk of melanoma, should seek to ensure vitamin D sufficiency."

This also explains one of the mysteries to arise from Australia and New Zealand. At this current time in planetary history, the southern hemisphere is – because of Earth's tilt angle – closer to the sun during summer than the northern hemisphere is during the northern summer. That means the southern nations are getting a stronger dose of UV radiation each year than Americans or Europeans.[256] It's one of the reasons that the antipodes share the highest rates of melanoma in the world. Yet here's the strange thing: they don't have the highest death rates from melanoma. Far from it.

This apparent contradiction was one of the first clues that led researchers to suspect vitamin D had a protective role against dying from cancer. How else could one explain the highest rates of melanoma in the world yet also the best survival rates?

---

256   Peak UV levels in New Zealand and Australia are 40% higher than peak levels in the UK or North America, according to the official position statement on UV and cancer published by the New Zealand Government's Ministry of Health

For inquisitive scientists like Leeds University's Julia A. Newton-Bishop – the lead author on the original study, these paradoxes opened up fresh grounds for investigation. If sunbathers were more likely to survive melanoma, could it possibly be that sunbathing might actually help prevent melanoma from developing in the first place?

The idea seems ludicrous – we all know that sunbathing causes melanoma, don't we? The reality is, we know less about the complex causes of melanoma than the simple messages published via the news media each summer imply.

Newton-Bishop's team continued to dig deeper for answers and, in late 2010, they made a bombshell discovery: British residents who sunbathed for five hours or more without sunscreen per day each weekend during summer reduced their risk of developing melanoma by an incredible 33%, compared with people who stayed out of the sun.

That's another of those let-it-sink-in moments.

If you look at it another way, people who obeyed the 'sun smart' message, slopped on the sunscreen and stayed out of the light, were a staggering 50% more likely to develop melanoma than people who actively sunbathed without sunscreen. This too might explain why so many melanoma victims in the media say, "but I only sunbathed occasionally, and I always tried to use sunscreen, it only took one time…".

"When the data were analysed for tumours in different body sites," reported the *European Journal of Cancer* study, "the protective effect of increased weekend sun exposure was strongest for limb tumours and tumours on rare body sites [those melanomas that frequently pop up where the sun don't shine]."

Sun-shy people had more than double the risk of developing head and neck melanomas than their tanned, beach-going compatriots.[257]

Which brings us back to the issue raised at the start of this chapter: why are those people who religiously use sunscreen the most likely to develop the deadliest skin cancer? The answer appears to lie in a battle between Nature and Big Pharma.

If you adhere to the 'nature' argument, humans have been living naturally under the sun for tens of thousands of years. Indeed, all life on earth is dependent on solar radiation and our bodies are highly attuned to deal with it. Why then, are we dealing with a sudden explosion in the number of skin cancer cases?

In humankind's quest to tame Nature, and indeed to advance ourselves, we have moved from a simple agricultural outdoors lifestyle to a mostly indoors one, particularly within the past 100 years. We no longer

---

257   A cautionary note. The protective effect of sunbathing did not extend to people with freckles, or photo sensitive skin. A common sense approach suggests vitamin D supplements are a better bet for those individuals.

spend long hours each day outside in the sun, developing protective suntans that last year-round. Instead, we creep from house to car to office to car to house, five days a week, barely getting a few minutes of genuine sun a day, if that.

As a result of our indoor lives, we find we now need protection from the sun because we don't have the time to build up tans gradually and naturally in the daylight in time for the summer break, we are simply too busy. So we reach for a pharmaceutical solution, trusting that the chemists have got it right and that human intelligence has beaten Nature.

This scenario would be all well and good – if sunscreens worked. The truth is, however, they have a lot of limitations. If your chances of getting melanoma were one in 1500 in 1935 (before the invention of sunscreens), and as high as one in 33 now, something has clearly gone wrong with the Big Picture.[258] In losing the protective effect of a long-lasting suntan, we have placed our trust in imperfect chemical formulations.

And here's where it went wrong. For decades, sunscreens were quite good at blocking UVB radiation, but utterly useless at blocking UVA radiation, which

---

258   In the interests of balance, it is worth pointing out that our sun has been more active over the past century than in the previous one thousand years. That was announced by the Max Planck Institute for Solar System Research in Germany in 2004 and reported in *The Telegraph*, 19 July 2004.

actually makes up nearly 95% of the total UV light reaching the surface of the earth. UVA penetrates glass (and sunglasses, incidentally), which UVB doesn't, and it penetrates more deeply into the human skin and so "may have greater destructive potential". It's known that UVA is more likely to age your skin and cause wrinkles. It is UVA that fades your carpets. UVB, on the other hand, is primarily responsible for causing sunburn but will also cause photo-aging of your skin.

However, here's the important part. It is UVB that primarily stimulates your body to produce more melanin, the darker protective pigmentation we call a suntan. UVA radiation will also create an instant same day tan, but it uses *existing* melanin in the skin to achieve this and thus doesn't actually stimulate a protective tanning response because it does not generate new melanin. This is one of the criticisms of sunbeds, which are mostly UVA driven – they're very good at creating a rapid tan, but the tan is not a protective one. You cannot take a sunbed tan out into the great wide open and assume you are protected.

So here's the twist. Sunscreens that blocked UVB actually prevented your body from defending itself from total solar radiation. Many of the melanomas appearing in Baby Boomers and Gen-X today are arguably a direct result of dodgy sunscreen products from the sixties onwards that gave people a false sense of security. They were doing more damage to themselves by lying in the sun all day with a UVB sunblock on, mistakenly believing that because they were not burning then they were safe. In the meantime, UVA radiation poured into them utterly unmolested.

"UVA may have a greater potential for carcinogenesis", reports the *Cleveland Clinic Journal of Medicine*.[259]

If this was an episode of *Star Trek*, a UVB sunblock while sunbathing (thus fooling the body into not generating a protective tan) is the equivalent of leaving the Enterprise "shields down" and unarmed while the enemy UVA sneaks aboard.

That, then, was strategic error number one. "A common misperception is that sunscreens decrease the risk of burning and allow people to increase their exposure to UV radiation. This results in increased exposure to UVA and thus increases the risk of skin cancers and facilitates photo-aging."[260]

Hands up everyone who has languished on the beach for hours, thinking that their sunscreen is protecting them.

For that reason, the industry has moved predominantly to "broad spectrum" sunscreens that claim to block both UVB and UVA rays. For those who regularly apply broad spectrum SPF-16 or higher every day, studies have shown a long term 38% reduction in the

259   "UV Protection and Sunscreens", Jou et al, *Cleveland Clinic Journal of Medicine*, Vol. 79, No. 6, June 2012

260   Ibid, sub-referencing "Sunscreen abuse for intentional sun exposure" by Autier, P. *Br Journal of Dermatology* 2009; 161(suppl 3):40-45

incidence of squamous cell carcinoma – one of the least harmful kinds of skin cancer.[261]

Sadly, that might be all that sunscreens do.

"Although sunscreens appear to be effective in preventing actinic keratosis [sun spots on the skin] and squamous cell carcinoma, the evidence that they also prevent basal cell carcinoma and melanoma has been inconclusive," reported researcher Paul Jou in June 2012.

Melanoma is the real killer when it comes to skin cancer. The mortality rate from melanoma is as high as one in five (20%). In contrast, the mortality rates from basal cell carcinoma (the most common skin cancer) and squamous cell carcinoma are around 1 in 333 (a 0.3% mortality rate). Melanoma is responsible for 75% of all skin cancer deaths. To discover that the primary weapon in the fight for a summer lifestyle is largely useless against the most common and deadliest skin cancers is disconcerting, to say the least.

A study from 2011 made the same point:[262]

"Safety of sunscreens is a concern," reports study author Dr Marianne Berwick, of the University of New Mexico's Cancer Centre and Department of Internal Medicine. "Sunscreen companies have emotionally and

261   "Prolonged prevention of squamous cell carcinoma of the skin by regular sunscreen use", Van der Pols et al, *Cancer Epidemiol Biomarkers Prev* 2006;15:2546-2548

262   "The Good, the Bad, and the Ugly of Sunscreens," M Berwick, Clinical Pharmacology & Therapeutics, Jan 2011, doi:10.1038/clpt.2010.227

inaccurately promoted the use of sunscreens."

With global sunscreen sales in the multi-billions of dollars every year, there's money to be made in selling products that can be linked to public health campaigns. The problem for consumers and regulators is whether in fact sunscreens are worth what we are paying for them, or whether consumer fears have been overhyped.

More disturbing in my view, however, is that sunsmart promotions are not passing on this inconvenient truth to the public. New Zealand's Cancer Society, for example, which as we've seen operates a very lucrative business in that country selling its own brand of sunscreen lotions, implies on its website that sunscreen protects against melanoma:

"New Zealand has the highest rate of melanoma in the world, and other skin cancers are also very common. You can help reduce your risk of skin cancer by using sunscreen the right way."[263]

If New Zealand's Cancer Society didn't have the reputation of a major medical charity to save them, they'd probably be at risk in my view of a false or misleading advertising prosecution – especially given the deadly impact of the claims.

---

263   "Sunscreen plain English Questions and Answers, 14 February 2012" NZ Cancer Society pamphlet, http://www. cancernz.org.nz/assets/files/info/SunSmart/Sunscreen%20 QA%27s_14Feb2012%283%29.pdf

Similar claims are made in Australia: "Skin cancer is one of the most preventable cancers, yet Australian adolescents have by far the highest incidence of malignant melanoma in the world," a spokeswoman for Sunsmart Australia said in a recent news release.[264]

On the basis of the science above, why are health agencies continuing to make these statements?

An Australian study often quoted by supporters of sunscreens was published in 2011.[265] It looked at an initial five year trial period and then a 10 year follow up, and found that regular users of broad spectrum sunscreens were less likely to develop primary melanomas. Critics, however, remain unconvinced.

"The study had serious limitations: the authors admitted that the results were marginally statistically significant; intervention sites of sunscreen application were chosen for nonmelanoma skin cancer and excluded the trunk and extremities, where melanomas often occur; and the entire body was analysed for melanomas, not just the intervention site. Thus, despite providing some of the first evidence supporting sunscreen's ability to prevent melanoma, these results are controversial and by no means conclusive."[266]

264   "Dark Side of Tanning Campaign conveys deadly message to young Victorians this summer", Sunsmart Australia news release, 2 December 2010

265   "Reduced Melanoma after Sunscreen Use", Green et al, *Journal of Clinical Oncology*, 2011; 29:257-263

266   "UV Protection and Sunscreens etc", Jou et al, citing a follow

In addition, a follow-up analysis published in the same journal working from the same Australian data actually found a *higher* rate of melanomas on areas that had been allegedly 'protected' by broad spectrum sunscreen.

You'll recall the studies quoted earlier where schoolchildren who used sunscreen regularly in controlled studies were actually more likely to develop melanoma precursors. The reason for this can possibly now be seen in context. By building a sun-safety message anchored primarily in the need for pharmaceutical companies to make a buck out of sunscreens, we have created a false but widespread public belief that sun exposure is easily controlled through sunscreens. It just isn't true. There are screeds of studies that prove sunscreens are effective at protecting against ageing of the skin, and against largely harmless forms of skin cancer. But let's face it, the real reason most people slop on the sunscreen is because they fear the Big-M that the media constantly warn them about.

So what happens when people swap their natural defence against melanoma (a suntan), for a solution obtained from a bottle that turns out to be ineffective? Melanoma rates go up despite increasing usage of sunscreens, and that's exactly what has happened since 1935.

---

up response, "Increased Melanoma After Regular Sunscreen Use?", Goldenhersh & Koslowsky, *Journal of Clinical Oncology*, 2011, 29:e557-e558

The weight of scientific evidence overwhelmingly suggests sunscreens don't protect you from melanoma and, worse, may actually increase your risk of developing it. In addition, because sunscreens are so good at blocking the vitamin D producing UVB rays, they may actually be seriously increasing your risk of dying from melanoma if you do develop it, because your body now lacks D's cancer-fighting protection.

Some of the same pharmaceutical companies who sold you the ineffective sunscreen in the first place will also make money from the hugely expensive cancer drugs or other medication you might later need.

It gets worse, however. You'll recall that sunscreens have an SPF factor, supposedly to reassure you of their relative strength and duration of protection. What most people don't know is that the SPF relates only to UVB radiation, not UVA. That means your SPF30+ sunscreen "might" give you all day protection from UVB (if applied under laboratory conditions), but it's doing nothing of the sort against deadly UVA rays.

"But they're all broad-spectrum sunscreens now, aren't they?" you ask. Only to a point: studies have shown that titanium dioxide, the most effective block against UVA known to man, was only able to muster up a protection factor of 12 for UVA radiation when used as directed in a recent experiment,[267] yet the same

267   "In vitro UV-A protection factor (PF-UVA) of organic and inorganic sunscreens", Couteau et al, *Pharmaceutical Development*

mineral managed to hit an SPF of 38 in another experiment. To draw an analogy, relying on a broad spectrum sunscreen to protect you from cancer-causing radiation is like playing Russian Roulette using a gun where four of the six chambers contain live bullets. And they don't tell you that on the back of the bottle.

Scientists actually don't know how much UVA is being blocked, and sunscreen manufacturers are arguing amongst themselves about the problem:

"To this day, SPF lotions vary greatly in their broad-spectrum protection," says a Procter & Gamble briefing. "Many SPF products claiming to reduce exposure to UVA do not even contain an FDA-recognized UVA sunscreen, such as avobenzone or zinc oxide."[268]

Now, here's the important bit:

"Currently, there is no universal test method or standard product label to indicate the level of UVA protection."

You read it right. We don't know how effective UVA sunscreens actually are. The labels on the bottle promise the earth, but it's unclear how much protection they are really delivering.

"Despite these variances in protection," reassures Procter & Gamble, "experts still agree that everyone should practice sun-safe strategies."

and Technology, 2009;14(4):369-72, http://www.ncbi.nlm.nih.gov/pubmed/19630696?dopt=Abstract

268   http://www.pgbeautyscience.com/assets/files/research_updates/UV%20Toolkit%20063005.pdf

California-based dermatologist Lawrence Samuels is another bemoaning the lack of hard and fast data on UVA protection:

"Unfortunately, at the present time there is no measure to quantify the effectiveness of a sunscreen's ability to block UVA rays. It is well known that chemical sunscreen ingredients that block UVA rays are somewhat unstable when exposed to UV rays and oxygen (air). This is further complicated by the fact that we do not have the ability to measure the stability or effectiveness of chemical sunscreens that block UVA rays."[269]

When you factor in that most of us don't use as much sunscreen lotion as manufacturers recommend, the protection factors (for what they're worth) will be lower again.

In other words, let the user beware. If you still think your sunscreen is truly a broad spectrum lotion protecting you from UVB and UVA radiation, you may be endangering yourself and your family. The effect of using a sunscreen that, at best, might only be shielding 25% of UVA radiation and 95% of UVB, is similar to being bombarded with UVA rays on a sunbed, which health officials are very vocal about, incidentally.

Further proof that natural tanners do better than sun-

---

269   "The Truth About Sunscreen and Effective Patient Education", Lawrence Samuels MD, *Practical Dermatology*, March 2011:27-32, http://www.bmctoday.net/practicaldermatology/pdfs/0311%20sunscreen%20feature.pdf

blockers comes from a 2009 study by the US Food and Drug Administration's Dianne Godar and others,[270] which found indoor office workers have higher melanoma rates than outdoor workers – a finding that supports Leeds University's Julia Newton-Bishop's conclusion that people who get outside in the sun at weekends are less likely to get melanoma than people who stay out of the sun.

"Paradoxically," reports Godar's study, "although outdoor workers get much higher outdoor solar UV doses than indoor workers get, only the indoor workers' incidence of cutaneous malignant melanoma (CMM) has been increasing at a steady exponential rate."

"The Godar paper argues that the environment we have created living indoors behind glass since the beginning of the 20th century, which allows exposure to UVA, but not UVB which synthesises vitamin D, is responsible for the epidemic of melanoma," explains Robert Scragg, a vitamin D expert at New Zealand's University of Auckland. Office buildings, homes and car windows have been allowing burning UVA radiation through while blocking UVB rays – which actually help generate protective vitamin D3 if they can reach your skin.

The US Food and Drug Administration study found

---

270   "Increased UVA exposures and decreased cutaneous Vitamin D(3) levels may be responsible for the increasing incidence of melanoma", Godar et al, *Medical Hypotheses*. 2009 Apr;72(4):434-43

vitamin D3 – created in the skin by suntanning – acts like a timebomb when it is absorbed by melanoma cancer cells.

"Outdoor exposures include UVB (290–320 nm) radiation, so that previtamin D3 and thermal conversion to vitamin D3 can occur in the skin. Vitamin D3 can then be converted to its most hormonally active form, 1a,25-dihydroxvitamin D3 or calcitriol, which kills melanoma cells and SCC (squamous cell carcinoma)," the Godar study reports.

The D3 attaches itself to melanoma cancer cells and explodes them.

"Calcitriol can control or eliminate melanoma cells by binding to the vitamin D3 receptor (VDR) on the nuclear membrane signalling for either growth inhibition or cell death via apoptosis, while it protects normal melanocytes from apoptosis."

Apoptosis is the way the body normally destroys cancer cells safely, but cancers spread when apoptosis isn't working properly. Vitamin D3 appears to power-up the body's natural cancer-destroying mechanisms.

We spend our working lives indoors, and the only times we go out in the sun we slap on a chemical cocktail capable of severely restricting vitamin D production.

Little wonder that an Austrian scientific study in the late nineties found users of sunscreens were a whopping three and a half times more likely to develop melanomas than regular unprotected sunbathers:

"The factor most significantly associated with increased melanoma risk was the use of sunscreens. Subjects who often used sunscreens had an increased odds ratio (OR) of 3.47 (95% confidence interval [CI]1.81-6.64) compared with subjects who never used sunscreens (P = 0.001), after adjustment for sex, age and other significant sunlight-related factors. Skin colour and higher numbers of sunbaths were significant protective factors."[271]

The Austrian team found that people who sunbathed more than 30 times a year reduced their risk of melanoma by a massive 91%. The only thing that ramped their risk right up again was if they got sunburnt doing it.[272]

A recent Swedish study, based on the knowledge that sunburn can lead to melanoma, examined society's most vulnerable – our children. Staggeringly,

271   "Phenotypic markers, sunlight-related factors and sunscreen use in patients with cutaneous melanoma: an Austrian case-control study", Wolf et al, *Journal of Melanoma Research*, 1998 Aug;8(4):370-8, http://www.ncbi.nlm.nih.gov/pubmed/9764814?dopt=Abstract

272   In contrast to the impact of sunbathing on reducing melanoma risk, the current 'darling' of dermatology is aspirin, with a number of reports suggesting low-dose aspirin daily can cut your risk of melanoma. If you read the following study, you'll see the risk reduction is 13% over a seven year period. Not quite a 91% risk reduction! See "Nonsteroidal anti-inflammatory drugs and the risk of skin cancer: A population-based case-control study," Johannesdottir et al, *Cancer*, online 29 May 2012, doi: 10.1002/cncr.27406

they found children whose parents regularly slopped sunscreen on them were more likely to get sunburnt:

"Sunscreen was an independent risk factor of being sunburnt between 2 and 7 years of age (not or seldom using sun screen was protective)... Swedish children are frequently sunburnt and children living in the south are more sunburnt than those in the north. Sunscreens that were seldom used or not used at all were found to be protective. These results support previous reports that photosensitive skin type is an important risk factor for suffering sunburn as a child and therefore increases the risk of cutaneous malignant melanoma."[273]

The Monty Python team could not have said it more deftly: "Sunscreens that were...not used at all were found to be protective".

In other words, parents who encouraged their children to tan naturally and gradually, without sunscreen, turned out to be more responsible than parents who followed official policy advice to slather on the sunscreen.

There are many scientists now daring to suggest that the sunscreen, sunsmart emperor has no clothes.

"Many primary care providers advise patients to use sunscreen as a means to reduce their risk for skin

---

273   "Factors related to being sunburnt in 7-year-old children in Sweden", Rodvall et al, *European Journal of Cancer*, 2010 Feb;46(3):566-72, http://www.ncbi.nlm.nih.gov/pubmed/19815405?dopt=Abstract

cancer, especially cutaneous malignant melanoma (CMM)," writes Dr Margaret Planta.[274] "Despite the availability and promotion of sunscreen for decades, the incidence of CMM continues to increase in the U.S. at a rate of 3% per year. There currently is little evidence that sunscreens are protective against CMM. A number of studies suggest that the use of sunscreen does not significantly decrease the risk of CMM, and may actually increase the risk of CMM and sunburns."

Planta warns "providers may need to alter their advice regarding sunscreen use for CMM prevention".

In 2006, the US Environmental Protection Agency put it on the record with a bald statement of fact, "there is no evidence that sunscreens protect you from malignant melanoma."[275]

Dr Planta cites more evidence, like the fact that residents of cooler northern US states like Delaware have a higher incidence of melanoma than sunnier southern states like Texas, which again suggests a greater and more regular sun exposure might actually protect against melanoma. Planta, incidentally, still insists sunscreens are necessary, but that the public need to be fully informed of their weaknesses.

---

274   "Sunscreen and Melanoma: Is Our Prevention Message Correct?", Margaret B. Planta MD, *Journal of the American Board of Family Medicine*, Nov-Dec 2011, vol 24 no. 6, 735-739 doi: 10.3122/jabfm.2011.06.100178

275   *United States Environmental Protection Agency. Sunscreen: The Burning Facts.* http://www.epa.gov/sunwise/doc/sunscreen.pdf.

"Future studies with humans," write Burnett & Wang in the conclusion of their own report, "will need to be conducted under real world conditions with modern sunscreens, before we can determine definitively the safety and efficacy of sunscreen.

"However, none of the data published to date *conclusively* demonstrate adverse effects on the health of humans from the use of sunscreens."

Dermatologists will frequently tell patients, "by the time you have a tan, the sun has already caused DNA damage inside you". Statements like this take a significant role in sunsmart messaging. However, whilst true, they are not the whole truth. Getting a tan is the body's response to UVB radiation – our DNA is actually programmed to repair the "damage" caused by UVB and to manufacture a protective tan as a result. *Without the damage, the DNA won't flip the switch to activate the tan.*

Further scientific evidence indicating that dermatologists may not have the full story emerged in a study published February 2012, in the journal *Mutation Research.*[276] Scientists discovered vitamin D actually

---

276   "Does vitamin D protect against DNA damage?," Nair-Shalliker et al, *Mutation Research*, 2012 May 1;733(1-2):50-7. See also "The Role of the Vitamin D Receptor and ERp57 in Photoprotection by 1α,25-Dihydroxyvitamin D3," Sequiera et al, *Molecular Endocrinology* February 9, 2012 me.2011-1161. See also "Vitamin D and skin cancer," Dixon et al, *Human Health Handbooks no. 1*, 2012, Volume 2, Part 5, 394-411, DOI: 10.3920/978-90-8686-

prevents DNA from being damaged by free radicals, and maintains genetic integrity. The vitamin also regulates the growth rate of cells and appears to "reduce oxidative damage in humans."

"Both animal studies and cell culture studies show that vitamin D treatment drastically reduced oxidative stress damage and chromosomal aberrations, and prevented telomere shortening and inhibiting telomerase activity, which also suggested that vitamin D may extend lifespan in humans," reported journalist David Liu of the findings.[277]

All of these things are what you would expect to find in a complex biological system where life has been reliant on the sun for millions of years. And so far, sun tans are looking a lot more protective against deadly skin cancers than anything humans have devised in the sunsmart arsenal. Maybe the natural response was the best after all.

After all, Cancer Research UK has announced "Over the last 25 years, rates of malignant melanoma in Britain have risen faster than any of the most common cancers." Melanoma's drag race up the fatality charts, then, has coincided with a similar mass uptake of sunscreens over the same period.

So what causes melanoma? A cynic at this point might be muttering "sunscreens", and for all we know

---

729-5_24

277 "Vitamin D may indeed help fight cancer," by David Liu, Food Consumer.org, 27 April 2012

that could be true. However, scientists have found some significant risk factors that point to whether you are more likely to develop melanoma.

They include:

- Fair skin (29% increase when compared against olive or brown-skinned people)
- Very fair skin (183% increase in risk)
- Blue/grey eyes (71% increase in risk compared with brown eyes)
- Green/hazel eyes (24% increase in risk)
- Blonde hair (76% increase in risk compared with black or brown haired people)
- Red hair (185% increase in risk)
- Able to get moderately tanned (31% increase in risk compared to people who easily tan deeply)
- Mild or occasional tans (88% increase in risk)
- No suntan at all, or freckled (124% increase in risk)

Additionally, your burn ratio is important. People who go brown without burning had no increase beyond the average risk, but for others:

- Mild burning followed by a tan (14% increase in risk)
- Painful sunburn followed by peeling (113% increase in risk)
- Severe sunburn with blistering (114% increase in risk)
- Sunburn before the age of 20 (24% increase in risk

compared with people never sunburnt)
- Sunburn since 20 (56% increase in risk)

The University of Leeds research unit discovered something else as well:

"We had known for some time that people with many moles are at increased risk of melanoma," Professor Julia Newton-Bishop explained, but "in this study we found a clear link between some genes on chromosomes 9 and 22 and increased risk of melanoma. These genes were not associated with skin colour."[278]

It was the first time science had found a genetic link to melanoma that did not involve hair, eye or skin colour. In this case, the genes influenced the number of moles a person has, and hence the number of pre-existing stepping stones that melanoma could spring from. The study determined that at least five genes exist that have an impact on melanoma risk, and most people in the world are carrying at least one of these genes. If you happen to be the lemon in the one-armed-bandit lottery and find you are carrying all five genes, your risk of developing melanoma is 800% higher than a person carrying none.[279]

---

278 "Moles and melanoma – researchers find genetic links to skin cancer", news release from Leeds Institute of Molecular Medicine and the Cancer Research UK Centre, 6 July 2009

279 In late 2011, the same research team uncovered three more genes adding to the risk. One DNA fault is linked to narcolepsy (suddenly falling asleep), the second is a faulty gene that fails to

Here's something else to think about: if you live in a high UV area like Queensland, sunburn easily or get skin cancer, which has a tiny mortality rate, a new study out of Australia indicates your risk of then developing pancreatic cancer (mortality rate 95% within a year, the remaining 5% soon after) is cut in half.[280] Most people survive breast cancer. The vast majority survive skin cancer. But you don't walk away from pancreatic cancer.

More people die each year from pancreatic cancer than skin cancer, it is the world's fourth most deadly cancer measured by number of deaths. Recent high profile victims include Apple co-founder Steve Jobs and actor Patrick Swayze. If it was likely that sunbathing would *increase* your risk of skin cancer, but *reduce* your risk of pancreatic cancer by 49%, how would you weigh your relative risk on this?

Tough question, but it's the kind we need to be asking ourselves because we don't live in a perfect world, and everything involves a trade-off of some kind.

There's something else about the pancreatic cancer study

repair damaged DNA in cells as it should, and the third risk factor is in a faulty gene that is supposed to prevent cancerous cells from spreading. If you are carrying all three of these gene faults, your risk of developing melanoma in your life is one in 46. See "Genome-wide association study identifies three new melanoma susceptibility loci", Barret et al, *Nature Genetics* [doi: 10.1038/10.1038/ng.959]

280   "Sun sensitivity linked to decreased pancreatic cancer risk, study suggests," Amanda Chan, *Huffington Post*, June 20, 2012, http://www.huffingtonpost.com/2012/06/20/sun-pancreatic-cancer-risk-sensitivity-uv-rays-vitamin-d_n_1609095.html

that's confusing researchers: is it vitamin D lowering the risk in this case, or is it sunlight itself? The implications of that are that there may be something protective in the way the human body processes UV radiation that mere vitamin D supplements can't replicate.

Their logic for saying this is that areas with the highest UV radiation in Australia have the lowest rates of pancreatic cancer, but that some studies have found no impact of vitamin D on this particular cancer.

Then there's another interesting revelation: sunburn might not be the cause of melanoma, merely an indicator that you are prone to melanoma. It seems like an odd thing to say, but a recent study reported:[281]

"Unfortunately, some aspects of the promotion and analysis of sunscreen use are controversial. Many take the perspective that if sunburns are strongly associated with the development of melanoma, and sunscreens prevent sunburn, then sunscreens will prevent melanoma.

"However…it is likely that sunburn is a clear indicator of the interaction between excessive sun exposure and a susceptible phenotype – that is, severe solar exposure to skin unaccustomed to it – rather than a direct cause of melanoma and basal cell carcinoma."

In other words, it is not that the sunburn necessarily causes the cancer, it's just that people most susceptible

---

281   "The Good, the Bad, and the Ugly of Sunscreens," M Berwick, *Clinical Pharmacology & Therapeutics*, Jan 2011, doi:10.1038/clpt.2010.227

to skin cancer burn more easily.

What then, can we take away from all this?

1. That sunscreens are excellent at helping prevent solar aging of the skin, and squamous cell carcinomas.

2. That there is currently no evidence that sunscreens are of any use at all in the fight against deadly skin cancers like melanoma and basal cell carcinoma.

3. That there is evidence people who regularly use sunscreen are paradoxically at a much higher risk of developing melanoma.

4. That if you sunburn easily or fall into a melanoma risk group (fair skin, blue or green eyes etc), it is very important that you do not sunburn.

5. That sunbathing without sunscreen during summer, but importantly also without burning, confers greater protection against melanoma than using sunscreen, but that this benefit does not exist for high risk individuals, who should use vitamin D supplements rather than sunlight.

6. That, used correctly, sunscreens make it impossible for your body to absorb healthy amounts of vitamin D.

7. That, seeing as most people don't use sunscreens correctly, those users are still getting some, if not the optimum amount, of vitamin D in summer.[282]

---

282   It is not true to claim, as some do, that slip, slop, slap has

The inconvenient truth about sunscreens, melanoma and cancer generally appears to be this: there is no easy solution. If you want youthful radiant skin, the price of beauty appears to be a much higher risk of breast, colon or other cancers of the internal organs, heart disease, Alzheimer's, multiple sclerosis, mental illness or a range of other nasties we've covered off in this book.

In short, it's a trade-off. The less sunlight you get, the happier your dermatologist will be, but the wealthier your oncologist, cardiologist and psychotherapist might become.

So what if you are one of those people who burns easily or who – despite what you've read here about the natural benefits of UV – doesn't want to spend time in the sun – how do you get sufficient vitamin D? As we're about to see, there are some alternative options.

---

not impacted vitamin D levels, as this snippet from a bowel cancer study illustrates: "Our findings are consistent with a recent analysis of the National Health and Nutrition Examination Survey (NHANES), which found a low mean plasma 25(OH)D level of 24 ng/mL among 13,369 participants between 2001 and 2004. This represented a marked decrease from NHANES III (1988 to 1994), when the mean 25(OH)D level was 30 ng/mL. Potential explanations for the rise in vitamin D insufficiency include increasing use of sunscreen for skin cancer prevention, decreased outdoor activity, and the rising prevalence of obesity." See http://jco.ascopubs.org/content/29/12/1599.full

Chapter 15

VITAMIN D: BEST SOURCES

"A wide range of epidemiologic and laboratory studies combined provide compelling evidence of a protective role of vitamin D on risk of breast cancer"
— *Dermato-Endocrinology Journal*, 2012

How much vitamin D should we consume? How much is poisonous? Where do we get it?

To answer the questions, we first have to understand the process. Food supplies only a limited amount of vitamin D.

"Unless those diets are rich in wild-caught fatty fish, sun dried Shitake mushrooms or wild reindeer meat," you can forget about "adequate" vitamin D intake from a healthy diet, says the Vitamin D Council's Dr John Cannell.

To get to 2,000IU a day through food alone, you would need to eat 50 eggs a day, or nine 1kg blocks of Swiss cheese, or 2kg of salmon. Anything less than that is playing.

The only food that comes close to giving you a decent vitamin D hit is sun-dried mushrooms. Shitake are the best to use, although you can use button or flat browns. Mushrooms, like humans, manufacture vitamin D when sunlight hits them. It's not the D3 variety that's best for us, but vitamin D2, created by plants and known as ergocalciferol. It is not quite as efficiently processed by our bodies, and most reports of vitamin D toxicity have arisen from being prescribed this vegan form of vitamin D2.

Where vitamin D3 is stored in our bodies for weeks, vitamin D2 is processed in hours or days.

However, here's the news. A hundred grams of mushrooms left to dry gills-up on the back porch in the summer sun for six hours a day, two days in a row, will create somewhere in the region of 46,000 units of vitamin D2 per 100 grams of mushroom. If you dry enough of them, and store them well, you'll have a weekly vitamin D2 hit available through winter.[283]

In Western Australia, commercial mushroom growers have cottoned onto this and are about to put vitamin D2 enhanced button mushrooms into supermarkets at the time of writing. They're using large, powerful UV lights to run their mushrooms under, and the growers say three button mushrooms will provide the recommended daily intake of vitamin D for Australians.

---

283   "Place mushrooms in sunlight to get your vitamin D: part one," Paul Stamets, *Huffington Post*, 2 July 2012

"It takes just two to three seconds for the mushrooms to generate an amount of vitamin D in excess of the daily recommended intake," reported a food industry paper.[284]

It's a good way of turning a public health issue into a daily meal marketing opportunity.

By far the biggest source of vitamin D, however, is solar.

If you sunbathe for half an hour, you will generate somewhere between 20,000 and 30,000 IU of vitamin D. That's the upper limit. After you reach those levels, the skin allows the excess vitamin D to be broken down by further sunlight. In other words, the body creates and stores as much as it needs, and no more.

To get that 20,000IU from your diet in half an hour, you would have to eat either forty servings of salmon, drink between 200 and 500 glasses of D-fortified milk (different countries fortify at different levels), or swallow twenty 1,000IU supplement pills. Obviously, that isn't going to happen.

The stores of vitamin D your body builds over summer and autumn are needed to carry you through winter, but by mid winter they'll have been used up, leaving you at the mercy of disease, which often hits hard in the winter and spring seasons.

As you've read in this book, many studies have shown

---

284   "Western Australia gets vitamin D enhanced mushrooms," 6 July 2012 www.freshplaza.com/print.asp?id=97180

a strong beneficial effect from higher daily doses (2000 to 4000IU) than are officially recommended.[285] While government health regulators drag their heels over boosting vitamin D levels, the public and their GPs are frequently taking matters into their own hands. But even then, without a good baseline of vitamin D, you may not be getting the full advantage.

"Very few humans obtain enough vitamin D even if they take several thousand units per day," warns researcher John Cannell. He cites a study of Hawaiian sunbathers which compared their vitamin D levels to a group of breastfeeding mothers being given 6,400IU in daily supplements. The study found that even mothers receiving that much vitamin D were using so much of it for their daily metabolism that almost none was being stored to fight diseases and boost immunity.[286]

"This implies virtually everyone has a chronic [vitamin D] deficiency, at least in the winter," says Cannell. "Because of this, most individuals have chronic substrate starvation, functional vitamin D deficiency, and thus, perhaps, higher risk for the 'diseases of civilisation'."

---

285   The Institute of Medicine lists these levels as "safe", but the RDI is set much lower

286   This also goes to the "breast is best" feeding argument. It is, but only if the mother has the proper reserves in her system of vitamin D. A 500IU dose from a pregnancy vitamin is not going to protect your baby or you. Breastfed babies are now a recognised risk group for vitamin D deficiency and rickets.

The problem can be expressed in laptop battery terms. Summer sun is like a full overnight charge for your computer battery. Daily supplements are like the trickle charge your battery receives while you use the laptop with the power cord plugged in. If your battery is low charged and you pull the cord out, it will go flat rapidly.

Think about that for a moment. If you don't build up good vitamin D stores in summer, or through some other means, even high daily supplements are not doing as much for your health as they could. Sure, they are better than nothing, but that's one of the reasons it is hard to turn your back on sunlight. It is impossible to overdose on vitamin D generated through UV rays, but it is possible to overdose on vitamin D taken orally.

Health authorities have sent out messages to medical practitioners urging them not to order blood tests for vitamin D deficiency because they are expensive, at around $50 to $100. Better, and cheaper, say the health agencies, simply to supply a prescription, no questions asked.

The only problem with that logic is that if your doctor doesn't know what your vitamin D levels actually are, how do they know what levels of the vitamin to give you for storage, and then how much to give you for daily maintenance? International research indicates a patient should be tested twice. Once in early spring to find their lowest vitamin D levels, and once in late summer for their peak level.

In New Zealand, for example, the standard medical prescription is a pill offering 50,000IU a month – roughly equivalent to sunbathing for 30 minutes twice in two days. Taken over a month, it averages out at a dose of around 1,500IU a day which, when you compare against the 6,400IU per day given to the breastfeeding women, is nothing. The mothers failed to store much of that 6,400 to fight cancers, so how much of the 1,500IU prescription dose will go to recharging batteries? Not a lot.

As if to prove the point, one study that gave vitamin D deficient patients 50,000IU a week for four weeks, and then 50,000IU a month for a year, managed to boost blood levels from 11 ng/ml at the start to 30 ng/ml by six months, and that's basically where it stayed for the rest of the trial, despite the seemingly large doses

It's the surplus amounts of vitamin D in your system, after basic bodily functions are taken care of, that are seized by the various vitamin D receptors (VDRs) throughout your organs and used to protect you, which is why the health effects of vitamin D can be seen on a sliding scale. People with blood levels of 30 ng/ml do better than people on 20 ng/ml, but people with enough vitamin D for 50ng/ml do better than all of them.

"If enough 25(OH)D substrate is available, multiple tissues are free to autonomously produce and locally regulate the amount of steroid needed for any particular disease state," says John Cannell.

"The fact that 20,000IU vitamin D can be produced in the skin in 30 minutes of sun exposure, combined with vitamin D's basic genomic mechanism of action, raises profound questions.

"Why did nature develop a system that delivers huge quantities of a steroid precursor after only brief periods of sun exposure? Would natural selection evolve such a system if the remarkably high input that system achieved were unimportant?"

Most people who manage to achieve the ideal 50-70 ng/ml of vitamin D in their blood have only done so through relying on UV rays, aided and abetted with high supplementation in the colder months.

Cannell's researchers estimate that a 1000IU daily supplement will boost your blood levels by about 10 ng/ml over a period of three months, so an average adult taking 2,000IU should be able to go from 10 to 30 ng/ml over that time. However, moving further up the range the increases are not linear, and if you begin with a baseline of 30 it might require higher amounts to reach 50 ng/ml than 2,000IU.

A study of middle-aged Canadians given supplements of 4,000IU a day for six months managed to punch their average blood levels up to 44 ng/ml with no side effects.[287] Another study shows healthy adult men can

---

287   "Randomised comparison of the effects of the vitamin D adequate intake vs 100mcg (4000IU) per day on biochemical responses and the wellbeing of patients," Vieth et al, *Nutrition* 2004;

usefully convert 5,000IU a day of vitamin day.[288]

"With regard to safety, sunlight is superior to oral supplementation," writes researcher Carol Wagner.[289] "One does not become vitamin D toxic from sunlight exposure; however, in comparison, people have become toxic from ingesting too much oral vitamin D. In an adult, it appears that the upper limit of tolerability of vitamin D is a daily consumption of thousands of international units of vitamin D—above 10,000 IU/day.

"There is a safety mechanism in place with sunlight: sunlight-derived vitamin D triggers downregulation of certain enzyme systems and upregulation of others in the body to dispose of any vitamin D and its metabolites not needed by the body. Judicious sunlight exposure is not a clear cut entity; however, as too much sun exposure can lead to sunburn, photoaging, and skin cancer."

There are important reasons not to simply self-medicate, even if tempted. In an advisory to medical practitioners on how to prescribe vitamin D, John Cannell warns that an enzyme known as Cytochrome P-450 plays a key role in the body's usage of vitamin D. "Therefore, drugs dependent on cytochrome P-450

Nutr J. 2004; 3: 8.
Published online 2004 July 19. doi: 10.1186/1475-2891-3-8, see http://www.ncbi.nlm.nih.gov/pmc/articles/PMC506781/
288   "The vitamin D epidemic and its health consequences," Holick MF, *Journal of Nutrition* 2005; 135:2739S-2748S
289   http://www.mdpi.com/2072-6643/4/3/208/htm

enzymes – and there are many – may affect vitamin D metabolism." Cannell says some medications raise D-levels, and others drop them, so it's up to doctors to test blood frequently if patients are taking medicines and more than 2000IU of vitamin D a day.

As a rule of thumb, Cannell advises pregnant mothers to seek 5000IU of vitamin a day from their doctors, on the grounds that not only is the vitamin crucial for human development but also that animal testing (controlled human testing on this aspect cannot be done for ethical reasons) has shown that when pregnant animals are deprived of vitamin D, their offspring are left with permanent brain injury.[290]

For mothers who are breastfeeding, Cannell recommends 7000IU a day which researchers say is enough to maintain maternal vitamin D levels and provide enough for the baby. If women do not have optimal blood levels, breastfed babies will need a further 800IU in supplements per day.[291]

---

290   "Developmental vitamin D deficiency alters brain protein expression in the adult rate: implications for neuropsychiatric disorders," Almeras et al, *Proteomics*, 2007; 7:769-780. See also "Developmental vitamin D3 deficiency alters the adult rat brain," Feron et al, *Brain Res Bull* 2005; 65:141-148, and also "Vitamin D deficiency during various stages of pregnancy in the rat; its impact on development and behaviour in adult offspring," O'Loan et al, *Psychoneuroendocrinology* 2007; 32:227-234

291   "Vitamin D requirements during lactation: high-dose maternal supplementation as therapy to prevent hypovitaminosis D for both the mother and the nursing infant," Hollis et al, *American*

Existing baby milk formulas contain vitamin D, but Cannell says babies should be getting a further 400IU daily on top of what's already in the milk powder, and toddlers and young children should be supplemented with 1000IU to 2000IU daily all year around. Dosages of 2000IU a day have been ruled safe for children over the age of one.

Vitamin D can be toxic in high doses. How high? Well, the upper limits are still being tested. Whilst it's not considered desirable to routinely have blood levels above 100 ng/ml, that's a target you won't hit even if you sunbathe all summer and take ordinary supplements – most of us would be struggling to hit 50 ng/ml.[292]

In some parts of the world and for some individuals, vitamin D levels are so bad that doctors have delivered injections containing 600,000IU to elderly patients, successfully raising blood levels from a death's door rate of 2 ng/ml to 27 ng/ml over six weeks. A study in the *Australian Medical Journal* has recommended 600,000IU doses for the elderly each autumn to cover them over winter and spring.[293]

Journal of Clinical Nutrition, 2004; 79:717-726

292   Having said that, doctors have deliberately dosed multiple sclerosis patients to bring their blood levels to an average of 154 ng/ml, with no negative effects during the 28 week trial. See "Safety of vitamin D3 in adults with multiple sclerosis," Kimball et al, *American Journal of Clinical Nutrition* 2007; 86:645-651

293   "Annual intramuscular injection of a megadose of

In New Zealand, doctors have administered doses of 50,000IU a day for ten days to kick start patients' vitamin D storage, and found no ill effects: "This regimen provides a simple, safe and effective way of managing vitamin D deficiency. Its short-term nature may result in higher compliance than daily dosing regimens," reported the study.[294]

In late 2010, however, the US health bureaucracy weighed into the vitamin D debate with a controversial report[295] that many in the industry saw as far too cautious. It pre-dated many of the studies detailed in this book, so some of its arguments have now been superseded, but essentially its line of reasoning was this:

Vitamin D is of proven benefit to the musculo-skeletal system, and increased intake can be justified on that basis alone. In the meantime, while there is evidence of an association between vitamin D and a number of other issues like cancer and cardiovascular disease, not enough randomized controlled trials have been done, the hard evidence is not yet there.

Collectively, thousands of scientists and medical researchers at the cutting edge of vitamin D studies

cholecalciferol for treatment of vitamin D deficiency: efficacy and safety data," Diamond et al, *Med J Aust* 2005; 183:10-12

294   "Efficacy of an oral, 10-day course of high-dose calciferol in correcting vitamin D," Wu et al, *N Z Med J.* 2003 Aug 8;116(1179):U536. deficiency

295   http://www.iom.edu/Reports/2010/Dietary-Reference-Intakes-for-Calcium-and-Vitamin-D.aspx

fell off their perches in surprise. While they knew that more randomised trials were needed, they also knew that if something walked like a duck, looked like a duck and quacked like one, chances are it wasn't a sparrow. The research on vitamin D, they pointed out, is extremely strong in some cases.

It seemed, to many, as if politics was intruding into science.

Among the critics, Vitamin D Council executive director Dr John Cannell, who issued this statement:

> Today, the Institute of Medicine's Food and Nutrition Board has failed millions... 3:00 PM PST November 30, 2010
>
> After 13 years of silence, the quasi governmental agency, the Institute of Medicine's (IOM) Food and Nutrition Board (FNB), today recommended that a three-pound premature infant take virtually the same amount of vitamin D as a 300 pound pregnant woman. While that 400 IU/day dose is close to adequate for infants, 600 IU/day in pregnant women will do nothing to help the three childhood epidemics most closely associated with gestational and early childhood vitamin D deficiencies: asthma, auto-immune disorders, and, as recently reported in the largest pediatric journal in the world, autism. Professor Bruce Hollis of the Medical University of South Carolina has shown

pregnant and lactating women need at least 5,000 IU/day, not 600.

The FNB also reported that vitamin D toxicity might occur at an intake of 10,000 IU/day (250 micrograms/day), although they could produce no reproducible evidence that 10,000 IU/day has ever caused toxicity in humans and only one poorly conducted study indicating 20,000 IU/day may cause mild elevations in serum calcium, but not clinical toxicity.

Viewed with different measure, this FNB report recommends that an infant should take 10 micrograms/day (400 IU) and a pregnant woman 15 micrograms/day (600 IU). As a single, 30 minute dose of summer sunshine gives adults more than 10,000 IU (250 micrograms), the FNB is apparently also warning that natural vitamin D input – as occurred from the sun before the widespread use of sunscreen – is dangerous. That is, the FNB is implying that God does not know what she is doing.

Disturbingly, this FNB committee focused on bone health, just like they did 14 years ago. They ignored the thousands of studies from the last ten years that showed higher doses of vitamin D helps: heart health, brain health, breast health, prostate health, pancreatic health, muscle health, nerve health, eye health, immune health, colon health, liver health, mood health, skin health, and especially fetal health.

Tens of millions of pregnant women and their breast-feeding infants are severely vitamin D deficient, resulting in a great increase in the medieval disease, rickets. The FNB report seems to reason that if so many pregnant women have low vitamin D blood levels then it must be OK because such low levels are so common. However, such circular logic simply represents the cave man existence (never exposed to the light of the sun) of most modern-day pregnant women.

Hence, if you want to optimize your vitamin D levels – not just optimize the bone effect – supplementing is crucial. But it is almost impossible to significantly raise your vitamin D levels when supplementing at only 600 IU/day (15 micrograms).

Pregnant women taking 400 IU/day have the same blood levels as pregnant women not taking vitamin D; that is, 400 IU is a meaninglessly small dose for pregnant women. Even taking 2,000 IU/day of vitamin D will only increase the vitamin D levels of most pregnant women by about 10 points, depending mainly on their weight. Professor Bruce Hollis has shown that 2,000 IU/day does not raise vitamin D to healthy or natural levels in either pregnant or lactating women. Therefore supplementing with higher amounts – like 5000

IU/day – is crucial for those women who want their fetus to enjoy optimal vitamin D levels, and the future health benefits that go along with it.

For example, taking only two of the hundreds of recently published studies:

Professor Urashima and colleagues in Japan, gave 1,200 IU/day of vitamin D3 for six months to Japanese 10-year-olds in a randomized controlled trial. They found vitamin D dramatically reduced the incidence of influenza A as well as the episodes of asthma attacks in the treated kids while the placebo group was not so fortunate. If Dr. Urashima had followed the newest FNB recommendations, it is unlikely that 400 IU/day treatment arm would have done much of anything and some of the treated young teenagers may have come to serious harm without the vitamin D.

Likewise, a randomized controlled prevention trial of adults by Professor Joan Lappe and colleagues at Creighton University, which showed dramatic improvements in the health of internal organs, used more than twice the FNB's new adult recommendations.

Finally, the FNB committee consulted with 14 vitamin D experts and – after reading these 14 different reports – the FNB decided to suppress their reports. Many of these 14 consultants are either famous vitamin D researchers, like Professor Robert Heaney at Creighton or, as in the case of Professor Walter Willett at Harvard, the single best-known nutritionist in the world. So, the FNB will not tell us what Professors Heaney and Willett thought of their new report? Why not?

Today, the Vitamin D Council directed our attorney to file a federal Freedom of Information (FOI) request to the IOM's FNB for the release of these 14 reports.

Most of my friends, hundreds of patients, and thousands of readers of the Vitamin D Council newsletter (not to mention myself), have been taking 5,000 IU/day for up to eight years. Not only have they reported no significant side-effects, indeed, they have reported greatly improved health in multiple organ systems.

My advice, especially for pregnant women: continue taking 5,000 IU/day until your 25(OH)D is between 50–80 ng/mL (the vitamin D blood levels obtained by humans who live and work in the sun and the mid-point of the current reference ranges at all American laboratories).

Gestational vitamin D deficiency is not only associated with rickets, but a significantly increased risk of neonatal pneumonia, a doubled risk for preeclampsia, a tripled risk for gestational diabetes, and a quadrupled risk for primary cesarean section.

Today, the FNB has failed millions of pregnant women whose as yet unborn babies will pay the price. Let us hope the FNB will comply with the spirit of "transparency" by quickly responding to our Freedom of Information requests.

John Jacob Cannell MD, Executive Director

It didn't actually take long for deep and far reaching criticisms of the Institute of Medicines report to emerge especially since, as Cannell alluded to, it had been peer reviewed by leading vitamin D specialists and found wanting.

One of those peer reviewers, Creighton University's Robert Heaney, was lead signatory on a letter in the medical press tearing the IOM report apart, in the restrained fashion that medical professionals are used to:[296]

"The Commentary by Ross et al.,"[297] concerning the recent calcium and vitamin D recommendations of the Institute of Medicine (IOM) has the potential to be substantially misleading. First, the title ("What clinicians need to know") is incorrect. The focus of all recommendations from the Food and Nutrition Board

---

296   http://jcem.endojournals.org/content/96/1/53/reply

297   Ross AC, Manson JE, Abrams SA, Aloia JF, Brannon PM, Clinton SK, Durazo-Arvizu RA, Gallagher JC, Gallo RL, Jones G, Kovacs CS, Mayne ST, Rosen CJ, Shapses SA 2011 The 2011 report on dietary reference intakes for calcium and vitamin D from the Institute of Medicine: what clinicians need to know. *J Clin Endocrinol Metab* 96:53-58

is, as the text of the article states, "normal healthy persons". Those recommendations have no applicability for patients with disease, or for physicians attempting to prevent disease in at-risk populations. That distinction is something clinicians need to know.

"The Commentary also gives no hint of the substantial dissent which the recommendations have evoked from the vitamin D investigative community. The draft report had been submitted to external experts, and it is to be presumed that their findings were made available to the panel.

"While the details of these reviews are shrouded behind a pledge of secrecy, it is clear from the published comments of several of them that the review uncovered errors both factual and strategic/analytic. Some acknowledgement of this dissent would have been useful. One infers that there must also have been dissent within the panel itself, as one of its members was a co-author of Canadian guidelines[298] which specifically recommended cholecalciferol intakes approximately three times higher than the IOM. Thus, rather than being a settled issue, clinicians need to know that the IOM recommendations do not represent a consensus.

---

298   Hanley DA, Cranney A, Jones G, Whiting SJ, Leslie WD, Cole DEC, Atkinson SA, Josse RG, Feldman S, Kline GA, Rosen C 2010 Vitamin D in adult health and disease: a review and guideline statement from Osteoporosis Canada. CMAJ 182: [Epub ahead of print Sept 7, 2010.]

"There is not room here to recount the many factual errors in the IOM report, some described elsewhere.[299] But two in particular are, we judge, suggestive of how the panel approached evidence…"

What followed were highly-technical discussions laced with juicy phrases like "osteoid volume (OV/BV) above 1% for 25(OH)D > 32 ng/mL," or "Nevertheless the IOM panel accepted 20 ng/mL as the lower bound of normal, despite the fact that approximately half of the individuals between 20 and 32 had OV/BV values above 1% (and ranging up to 4.5%)…"

In the end, the accusation appeared to come down to one of politics:

"In both instances, there seemed to have been an effort to discredit or distort studies that were incompatible with the panel's proposed 20 ng/mL lower bound for normal vitamin D status.

"Finally, in their conclusion, Ross et al. call for more randomized controlled trials. This is such a part of the conventional wisdom that it would seem to be entirely reasonable. Instead it dodges the panel's responsibility to deal with the available evidence. Most of the "needed" randomized trials are simply unfeasible (8),

---

299   "Why the IOM recommendations for vitamin D are deficient," Heaney RP, Holick MF 2011. *J Bone Miner Res* (in press) March 2011 [Epub ahead of print 1/5/11.]
4. "The D-batable Institute of Medicine report: A D- lightful perspective," Holick MF 2011. *Endocr Prac* 17:143-149

as they would require low intake contrast groups with serum 25(OH)D levels below even the IOM's already low recommendation. Such trials would be unethical. Since they cannot be done, this purported "need" leaves critical nutritional policy issues in a kind of permanent limbo."

In medical science, 'them's fightin' words'.

Researcher Dr William Grant waded in, noting that the IOM had cherry-picked studies it liked, and ignored randomized controlled trials it didn't like, such as the ones you've read in this book:

"The committee appeared to have a bias of excluding RCTs on such outcomes as cancer and influenza incidence and effects during pregnancy that were not in line with its eventual recommendations," said Grant in a 2012 review.[300]

"This report has been severely criticized by the vitamin D research community, with over 125 journal publications to date disagreeing with the recommendations. A representative paper stated: 'The IOM recommendations for vitamin D fail in a major way on logic, on science, and on effective public health guidance. Moreover, by failing to use a physiological referent, the IOM approach constitutes precisely the wrong model

---

300   "Top Vitamin D Papers of 2011 – Dosage Recommendations and Clinical Applications," William B. Grant, Ph.D, April 10, 2012, http://orthomolecular.org/resources/omns/v08n12.shtml

for development of nutritional policy.[301]

"The case could be made that the IOM committee, by setting the recommended dose so unreasonably low, is putting the U.S. population at greatly increased health risk. Further, much of the rest of the world's countries look to the IOM report for guidance, placing a major portion of the world's population at risk."

Weighing up the Institute of Medicine's "prove it" position, researchers went back and tested the thousands of studies already done: Is there sufficient evidence already on the table to justify high-dose vitamin D as a preventative? Their conclusion: there is, and people probably shouldn't wait for official advice before acting.[302]

"A wide range of epidemiologic and laboratory studies combined provide compelling evidence of a protective role of vitamin D on risk of breast cancer. This review evaluates the scientific evidence for such a role in the context of the A.B. Hill criteria for causality, in order to assess the presence of a causal, inverse relationship, between vitamin D status and breast cancer risk.

"After evaluation of this evidence in the context of

---

301   "Why the IOM recommendations for vitamin D are deficient," Heaney RP, Holick MF.. *J Bone Miner Res.* 2011;26(3):455-7

302   "Does the evidence for an inverse relationship between serum vitamin D status and breast cancer risk satisfy the Hill criteria?", Mohr et al, *Dermato-Endocrinology*, Volume 4, Issue 2 April/May/June 2012, http://www.es.landesbioscience.com/journals/dermatoendocrinology/2012DE0186.pdf

Hill's criteria, it was found that the criteria for a causal relationship were largely satisfied.

"Studies in human populations and the laboratory have consistently demonstrated that vitamin D plays an important role in the prevention of breast cancer.

"Vitamin D supplementation is an urgently needed, low cost, effective, and safe intervention strategy for breast cancer prevention that should be implemented without delay. In the meantime, randomized controlled trials of high doses of vitamin D_3 for prevention of breast cancer should be undertaken to provide the necessary evidence to guide national health policy."

In June 2012 the Endocrine Society published its own statement on vitamin D, noting "strong association" between the vitamin and a range of health issues as outlined in this book. However, with a lack of randomised controlled trials in many areas, the Society could not step ahead of the evidence and make across the board recommendations.[303]

"Although future research may demonstrate clear benefits for vitamin D in relation to cancer and possibly support higher intake requirements for this purpose, the existing evidence has not reached that threshold.

"There is emerging evidence that vitamin D may directly regulate immune function, both innate and adaptive. However, it will require large well-designed

303   Rosen et al, *Endocrine Reviews*, June 2012, 33(3):456–492
http://edrv.endojournals.org/content/33/3/456.full.pdf+html

clinical trials to prove that vitamin D supplementation could enhance innate immunity or reduce the severity of autoimmunity.

"In summary, not surprisingly there remains a persistent need for large randomized controlled trials and dose response data to test the effects of vitamin D on chronic disease outcomes including autoimmunity, obesity, diabetes mellitus, hypertension, and heart disease."

The problem is, randomised controlled trials are expensive. Normally they are done by drug companies with a patented drug that they can then sell for billions under licence as part of recouping the research costs. Vitamin D on the other hand is non-patentable, natural and cheap. Pharmaceutical companies are not exactly falling over themselves to fund full vitamin D3 trials for two reasons. 1, they make no money. 2, if they prove that vitamin D3 does improve your health to the extent now believed by researchers, that could represent a massive fall in profits for pharmaceutical companies in the face of sliding demand for their medicines. Which may be the reason some in the medical establishment are dragging their heels on vitamin D as well.

There is also the reality, as you've seen in this book, that some randomized human trials would quite simply be unethical. We cannot starve a baby or a foetus of vitamin D in a double-blind trial. There are therefore considerable areas of research where we cannot push research to the nth degree, but only rely on observational studies after the fact.

Despite the crying need for randomised trials, few have been undertaken:

"The function and requirement of vitamin D during pregnancy for both mother and fetus have remained a mystery. This fact was highlighted by *The Cochrane Review* in 2000, which reported a lack of randomized controlled trials (RCTs) with respect to vitamin D requirements during pregnancy. Unfortunately, during the past decade only a single RCT has been performed with respect to vitamin D requirements during pregnancy."[304]

That study, incidentally, was performed by vitamin D researchers on their own initiative. The bottom line appears to be a simple choice: do we as members of the public begin boosting our vitamin D levels on the basis that it can't do any harm to bring them up to where nature expects them to be, or should we sit and wait for the health bureaucracy?

---

304   "Vitamin D and Pregnancy: Skeletal Effects, Nonskeletal Effects, and Birth Outcomes," Hollis & Wagner, *Calcified Tissue International*, 2012, DOI: 10.1007/s00223-012-9607-4

Chapter 16

THE NZ POSITION: A COMMENTARY

"The Ministry of Health says supplements
aren't necessary"

– NZ Listener, 2012

There are big discrepancies between what is regarded
as a deficient vitamin D intake and what is not. Deficiency was defined in the 2002 Children's Nutrition
Survey as less than 17.5 nmol/L of vitamin D in blood
(8 ng/ml),[305] whereas the international Vitamin D
Council would classify that as "seriously deficient".

The now internationally accepted "seriously deficient"
level of less than 25 nmol/L (10 ng/ml) is classified by
New Zealand authorities as only "moderately deficient", and even "deficient" doesn't kick in here until
it's below 17 nmol/L (7 ng/ml).[306] Is this Orwellian
newspeak or simply a reflection of the mental acuity

---

305   "Sun-shy infants developing rickets'", *NZ Doctor*, 14
December 2011
306   Ibid

of the Wellington health bureaucracy? It appears to be the latter.

Because New Zealand's Ministry of Health is still in denial after seven years about the benefits of vitamin D in fighting anything but rickets, it still defines vitamin D 'adequacy' in skeletal health terms, which is a strategic mistake.[307] Bones require much lower doses of vitamin D to maintain good bone health, meaning just because you have "adequate" vitamin D in that area, does not mean you have enough vitamin D to fight cancer or heart disease.

This jargon, in policy documents for doctors and the media, implies – whether intentionally or not – that New Zealand's vitamin D problem isn't all that bad. The New Zealand news media probably don't appreciate the subtle nuances in the jargon, and simply assume that when Ministry of Health says only 10% of New Zealand children are vitamin D "deficient", that this is based on an equivalent scale to that used overseas. Unfortunately, it is not.

Qatari health authorities, for example, say children with "less than 20 ng/ml vitamin D were deemed deficient", yet NZ bureaucrats call a level half that – 10 ng/ml – only "moderately deficient".[308]

---

307   Or possibly deliberate, given that the US Institute of Medicine has pulled exactly the same stunt.
308   "Vitamin D deficiency as a strong predictor of asthma in children," Bener et al, *International Archives of Allergy &*

It is as if you can pretend an epidemic does not exist by inventing your own definitions of deficiency that bear no relation at all to international best practice or the latest research data. In sunny Qatar they found 36% of children deficient in vitamin D. In cooler, cloudier New Zealand we're told only 10% of kids are "deficient".

Pressure from independent media reports on vitamin D in 2005, and again in early 2008, led to New Zealand's Ministry of Health and the Cancer Society issuing a joint position statement. Whilst acknowledging that sun exposure has benefits for vitamin D absorption, and recommending that people get sun exposure outside peak hours in summertime and during peak hours in winter, the two organisations ultimately threw their hands in the air and kicked for touch:[309]

"Vitamin D is a hormone with receptors located in organ tissues throughout the body. Recent research suggests possible beneficial effects of exposure to solar UVR in the prevention or improvement in outcome of treatment for a number of other diseases including breast, prostate and colorectal cancer, non-Hodgkin lymphoma, diabetes, autoimmune disease (eg, multiple sclerosis) and hypertension.

"Although vitamin D may be a contributing factor

Immunology, 2012; 157:168-175

309   "Position Statement: The risks and benefits of sun exposure in New Zealand", Cancer Society et al, August 2008

to disease risk reduction for these conditions, it is not clearly known whether there are factors, other than vitamin D, which may play an important role.

"There is insufficient evidence to assume that vitamin D supplementation and sun exposure are equivalent in their beneficial effects. Therefore, at this time, no definitive action can be taken on these findings nor any recommendations made, as further research is required."

That was 2008. Most of the studies you have read about in this book were published after that. A fair and reasonable reader might well say the jury is well and truly in. So it was with some surprise that in their revised position statement of 2012 the two agencies state:[310]

"A rapidly-growing body of evidence has identified an association between low vitamin D levels and non-skeletal health outcomes such as colorectal cancer, cardiovascular disease, auto-immune conditions and all-cause mortality, but so far there is no evidence of a causal role (Institute of Medicine 2011).

"In the absence of convincing evidence from inter-vention trials, there is no basis for their inclusion in public policy at present."[311]

---

310 "Consensus Statement on vitamin D and sun exposure in New Zealand," Ministry of Health and Cancer Society of New Zealand, 14 March 2012

311 One of the studies New Zealand authorities rely on for

So, based on the discredited thinking of the bureaucrats at the Institute of Medicine, New Zealand is still kicking for touch. Readers can judge for themselves whether the science quoted in this book is convincing enough to justify boosting their own vitamin D levels.

The Consensus Statement[312] still refuses to admit that its vitamin D intake recommendations are themselves "seriously deficient".

Most of the scientific and medical studies you've read have revealed a sliding scale of health benefits – the more vitamin D in the blood, the better the survival or immunity outcome. Some of the blood levels to achieve that have been as high as 80 ng/ml (200 nmol/L).

---

the "inconclusive" claim is the Women's Health Initiative study reported at the start of the Breast Cancer chapter in this book. Because of its size, involving more than 30,000 women, research teams keep dipping into it and proclaiming there's no link between vitamin D and cancer. But the data sample was fundamentally-flawed, in that the vitamin D dose of 400IU a day has since been shown to be too small to influence cancer. As one research team noted last year, rely on the WHI study at your peril: "The low vitamin D dose provided, limited adherence, and lack of serum 25(OH)D values should be considered when interpreting these findings." See "The Effect of Calcium plus Vitamin D on Risk for Invasive Cancer: Results of the Women's Health Initiative (WHI) Calcium Plus Vitamin D Randomized Clinical Trial", Brunner et al, *Nutrition and Cancer* Volume 63, Issue 6, 2011

312   Beloved of politicians and bureaucrats, "Consensus" is a dirty word in real science. Science works by continuous progression, testing and re-testing. Anything and everything is open to challenge, if it can be proven. "Consensus" is the last refuge of charlatans, because it implies the science is settled when it never can be.

Despite that, the Consensus report says:

"Some international policy statements on vitamin D have defined an adequate serum 25(OH)D level as 50 nmol/L [just 20 ng/ml] and over (Institute of Medicine 2011; American Academy of Dermatology and AAD Association 2010)...

"There is also variation in the use and definition of the terms 'adequate', 'sufficient' and 'optimal' due to a lack of evidence. Based on the knowledge available, it is not possible to determine an optimal status level, but aiming for a 25(OH)D level of 50 nmol/L or more seems prudent."

The politics behind it can be seen in the experts the Ministry of Health and the Cancer Society chose to quote in regard to "adequate" levels of vitamin D: "Institute of Medicine 2011; American Academy of Dermatology and AAD Association 2010".

There are thousands of scientists, doctors and medical researchers more qualified to comment on vitamin D adequacy than the Dermatology Association. The Institute of Medicine report received such a kicking from 14 vitamin D experts invited to peer review it that their criticisms were suppressed, which speaks volumes as to the IOM's integrity and the NZ Ministry of Health's reliance on it.

New Zealand's Ministry of Health would have you believe that only 4.9% of New Zealand adults are 'deficient' in vitamin D, and only 0.2% are 'seriously deficient'. A further 27.1% of adults in 2008 "were below recommended levels but did not have a deficiency".[313]

It is not until you read the New Zealand definitions that you see how dangerous such Orwellian Newspeak can be. While this book is full of peer reviewed scientific studies listing 'serious deficiency' as less than 10 ng/ml, New Zealand defines serious as 5 ng/ml or less. From 5 ng/ml to 9.99 ng/ml is defined in New Zealand as "mild to moderate deficiency". Again, in the rest of the civilised world this is all still seen as "serious deficiency".

From 10 ng/ml through to 20 ng/ml, New Zealand calls this "below recommended level but not deficient". I do hope my journalistic colleagues reading this now realise how badly the New Zealand Ministry of Health has conned them. As you've seen in this book, levels below 20 ng/ml are regarded as "deficient" everywhere else in the world. Even New Zealand scientists are using the internationally accepted definitions.[314]

So if we redefine the Ministry of Health propaganda, what we actually have is 5.1% of New Zealand adults who are 'seriously deficient', and a further 27.1% who

313   "Vitamin D Status of New Zealand Adults," Ministry of Health, 14 March 2012, http://www.health.govt.nz/publication/vitamin-d-status-new-zealand-adults

314   Auckland Hospital has been known to pump people with 50,000IU of vitamin D per day for 10 days in order to provide emergency boosts, after discovering vitamin D levels just under 10 ng/ml, http://www.ncbi.nlm.nih.gov/pubmed/14513083

are 'deficient', for a grand total of 32.2% of New Zealanders – one in three of us – who are deficient in vitamin D.

The average level of vitamin D, for all New Zealand adults, is only 25.2 ng/ml (63 nmol/L), meaning our national average is what the rest of the world calls "insufficiency".

One recent study out of the US involving cancer specialists[315] defines vitamin D levels in a way that makes New Zealand's Ministry of Health appear incompetent:

"A widely accepted classification is deficiency at <20 ng/ml [50 nmol/L], insufficiency at 20–31 ng/ml [50-77 nmol/L], and an optimal range of ≥32 ng/ml [80 nmol/L]."[316]

As for the claims that there are no firm scientific studies showing improvements for patients given vitamin D in controlled trials, well that's a load of old cobblers as well. Every day, reports like this one are making the news internationally:[317]

---

315   "The effect of various vitamin D supplementation regimens in breast cancer patients", Peppone et al, *Breast Cancer Research & Treatment*, Volume 127, Number 1 (2011), 171-177, http://www.ncbi.nlm.nih.gov/pmc/articles/PMC3085185/

316   "Vitamin D insufficiency in North America," Hanley et al, *J Nutr.* 2005;135:332–337 See also:
"Redefining vitamin D insufficiency," Malabanan et al, *Lancet.* 1998;351:805–806. See also: "Estimates of optimal vitamin D status", Dawson-Hughes et al, *Osteoporos Int.* 2005;16:713–716

317   "Vitamin D Deficiency And Lung Function In Asthmatic

A new study from researchers in Boston has found that poorer lung function in asthmatic children, treated with inhaled corticosteroids, is linked with vitamin D deficiency.

Ann Chen Wu, MD, MPH, assistant professor in the Department of Population Medicine at Harvard Medical School and Harvard Pilgrim Health Care Institute said:

"In our study of 1,024 children with mild to moderate persistent asthma, those who were deficient in vitamin D levels showed less improvement in pre-bronchodilator forced expiratory volume in 1 second (FEV1) after one year of treatment with inhaled corticosteroids than children with sufficient levels of vitamin D."

The study, which was published in American Journal of Respiratory and Critical Care Medicine, used data from the Childhood Asthma Management Program. It was a multi-center trial of asthmatic children between 5 and 12 years of age who were randomly assigned to treatment with nedocromil, budesonide (inhaled corticosteroid), or a placebo. The patients' vitamin D levels were categorized as deficient (≤ 20 ng/ml), insufficient (20-30 ng/ml), or sufficient (> 30 ng/ml).

Pre-bronchodilator FEV1 was increased during

Children," *Medical News Today*, 14 July 2012, http://www.medicalnewstoday.com/articles/247836.php

a treatment period of 12 months by 330 ml in the vitamin D insufficiency group that were treated with inhaled corticosteroids. In the vitamin D sufficiency group, kids with the same treatment saw a 290 ml increase, and in the vitamin D deficiency group only 140 ml increase.

In other words, asthmatic children with higher vitamin D found their medication was more than twice as effective as those with low vitamin D levels. It can't be true, of course, because the Ministry of Health and NZ Cancer Society say such intervention studies don't exist.

Sharp-eyed readers may have noticed that blood levels of 20 ng/ml (50 nmol/L) were deemed as "deficient" in the July 2012 Harvard study, yet that's the level the Ministry of Health hotshots are trying to convince New Zealanders is a good target to aim for. The level found to actually be "sufficient" in the asthma study is 75 nmol/L, well above the MoH target.

On the same day as the Harvard study, another news agency reported high vitamin D levels in breast cancer patients are linked to smaller tumours, while deficient levels of vitamin D led to larger tumours:[318]

---

318   "High vitamin D levels better breast cancer outcomes," by David Liu PhD, Food Consumer, 14 July 2012, http://www. foodconsumer.org/newsite/Nutrition/Vitamins/vitamin_d_breast_cancer_071410429.html

The benefits of vitamin D seemed particularly stronger among postmenopausal women with breast cancer. Among postmenopausal breast cancer patients, those with greater than 30 ng of vitamin D3 per mL of blood at diagnosis (75 nmol/L) were 85 percent and 57 percent more likely to survive from the disease and have disease-free interval, respectively, than those who had less than 30 ng per mL.

The study concluded high vitamin D levels at early breast cancer diagnosis are correlated with smaller tumor sizes and better overall survival odds, and improve breast cancer-specific outcome, particularly in postmenopausal patients.

The great thing about living in a free country is you can choose who you prefer to believe, the cancer specialists reporting in the journal *Carcinogenesis*, or the New Zealand Ministry of Health team telling you that 20 ng/ml of vitamin D (50 nmol/L) is perfectly fine and that even less than that is probably sufficient. Please bear in mind however that the MoH choose to receive their advice on adequate vitamin D levels from dermatologists and a sunscreen manufacturer.

It was a dermatologist who famously said, "science has never proven that a lack of vitamin D causes cancer."[319]

319   "Bikini parade raises eyebrows in Minnesota town," *Duluth News Tribune*, 18 July 2012

To be fair, though, many of the excellent studies quoted in this book have been done by dermatologists, and it's too easy to tar an entire profession over statements made by a few. British Association of Dermatologists spokeswoman Deborah Mason understands the issue well:

"Enjoying the sun safely, while taking care not to burn, can help to provide the benefits of vitamin D without unduly raising the risk of skin cancer. The time required to make sufficient vitamin D is typically short and less than the amount of time needed for skin to redden and burn. Regularly going outside for a matter of minutes around the middle of the day without sunscreen should be enough.

"When it comes to sun exposure, little and often is best, and the more skin that's exposed, the greater the chance of making sufficient vitamin D before burning."[320]

Speaking of sunscreen manufacturers, what of the Cancer Society, an organisation seeking millions of dollars in public donations every year? Cancer kills one in three New Zealanders, yet the needs of the many seem outweighed by the needs of the few and the powerful dermatology lobby group. It is also relevant, in my view, that the Society makes a substantial amount of money from the 'sunscare' business, particularly in light of massive questions about the safety and effectiveness of sunscreens.

---

320   "The power of D", *The Press & Journal UK*, 2 June 2012

In the meantime, thousands of people are dying of preventable disorders, while health bosses continue to focus on a minority cancer that kills only a few people each year, despite the vast numbers who develop it.

Perhaps what this controversial debate is really about is not skin cancer but ageing. Yes, UV radiation ages skin. In refusing to age gracefully and naturally, in maintaining our battle to retain our youth, we're now running a serious risk of not ageing at all – not living long enough to age. Staying young. Dying pretty. But dying, nonetheless.

The overseas, and indeed NZ, research laid out in this book has shown that New Zealand's official Recommended Daily Intake of only 200IU of vitamin D a day is laughable, ludicrous and decades out of date. Such tiny amounts might be enough to bring rickets under control, but they will do nothing to boost your immune system or lower the risk of heart attack, stroke or cancer. They will certainly do nothing to reduce the risk of autism or numerous other diseases.

A major New Zealand magazine nonetheless reported in April 2012 that only "very small amounts" of sun exposure are needed to gain protection, "but if you're worried, you can top up the levels in your diet: oily fish, egg yolks, margarine – cod liver oil if you must."[321]

The advice is just wrong, unless of course the maga-

---

321   "The Vitamin D Factor," by Jennifer Bowden, *NZ Listener*, 21 April 2012

zine really meant "wild-caught fatty fish, sun-dried Shitake mushrooms or reindeer meat," the latter being in somewhat of a short supply down under. The amount of New Zealand fortified milk a person would have to drink to get the 20,000IU dose equivalent to half an hour in the sun is 500 glasses. The patient would have drowned long before reaching that target.

"If that doesn't suit you," continues the cover story helpfully, "you could take over the counter supplements, although the Ministry of Health says supplements aren't necessary for people with no specific medical issue or risk factors."

Once again, terrible, even deadly advice. The whole point of vitamin D is to be the preventative at the top of the cliff, rather than the last chance medication at the bottom once you've already developed a serious illness.

This is the same Ministry of Health, however, that defines "deficiency" as less than 17.5 nmol/L (8 ng/ml). Contrast this statement from the latest Australian scientific study on deficiency: "Serum 25(OH)D levels of <50 nmol/L (20 ng/ml) were considered vitamin D deficient."[322]

New Zealand's Ministry of Health says only 5% of New Zealanders are "deficient". In sunny Australia

---

322   "25-Hydroxyvitamin D Levels and chronic kidney disease in the AusDiab (Australian Diabetes, Obesity and Lifestyle) Study," Damasiewicz et al, *BMC Nephrol.* 2012 Jul 3;13(1):55

they say its 31%.[323] Under my own reading of the NZ raw data against the Australian definition, 32.2% of New Zealanders are "deficient". Who is most likely to be right, here?

It's also the same Ministry of Health that tells journalists "there is no scientifically validated safe level of UV exposure", which sounds all serious and official until you wake up, pinch yourself, slap yourself for extra good measure, and realise the sun has been shining on humans since we first walked the earth, and that our bodies are designed to process UV radiation for the greater good of our health.

If MoH wants to be pedantic, "there is no scientifically validated safe level of exposure" either to the 20,000 pieces of man-made orbital space junk hanging above our heads 24/7, but somehow we survive and death by satellite is a relatively rare misadventure.[324]

Every breath we take brings us one step closer to death. Every move we make wears out cells and joints. I'm sure a case could be made that we should reduce taking breaths and stay locked inside a safe cocoon. Me? I prefer living.

To say that humans should avoid the sun is, frankly, unnatural, not to mention unscientific – flying as it

---

323   Ibid

324   "Will your home and your car be covered when the NASA satellite breaks up and falls to Earth later this week?" MSNBC, 19 Sept. 2011

does in the face of millions of years of live human trial evidence to the contrary. To say it with a straight face is pure, albeit unintentional, comedy gold. Chicken Little is well and truly in charge of the hen house.

It is probably time that New Zealand journalists attending Ministry of Health briefings on the vitamin D issue tested what they're being fed, lest they discover it is the food traditionally used to grow those aforementioned Shitake mushrooms.

New Zealand's official state of denial probably has more to do with the incredible power of the dermatology lobby in New Zealand's health system and the amount of taxpayer money that has been invested in slip, slop, slap at their urging. Cancer specialists, cardiologists, endocrinologists and GPs have largely figured this out now, and instead of fighting Wellington directly they're simply prescribing large vitamin D supplements and some regular sun as part of routine patient care.

Vitamin D is so cheap and available, and its benefits potentially so vast, that the results are likely to speak for themselves.

THE CRITICS ON *BREAKING SILENCE*:

"Breaking Silence is not on my recommended read list. I firmly believe it is *compulsory* reading for anyone over 18." – Andrew Stone, *Albany Buzz* business magazine

"The book has real value" – Larry Williams, Newstalk ZB

"I found it an incredibly surprising book, and a very relevant book, and a very important book". – Anna Smart, Newstalk ZB

"I had no particular views on the case before this book came out but I have to say it's a powerful read. An influential read, one might say... All those people who poured out their invective when it became known the book was about to hit the book shops really should just read it for themselves. It may not be quite what they think." – Helen Hill, *The Marlborough Express*

"Breaking Silence is a chilling narrative and the most important I have read. Adults may need to read the story to gain any understanding. Younger people should read in it a warning: that it is the way we make decisions early on that may determine the course of our life and the lives of those entrusted to our care." – Pat Veltkamp Smith, *Southland Times*

"The book so many maligned before it came out reveals a mother we haven't met. When I last wrote about Macsyna King, I said I didn't think I'd like her. I've changed my mind. I certainly think she out-classes the Wellington radio announcer who posted on Facebook that after receiving her advance copy of *Breaking Silence*, she had "spat on it, wiped my ass on it, and ripped it up". – Tapu Misa, *NZ Herald*

"Actually, the rumours of Wishart's death as an investigative journalist turn out to be greatly exaggerated. *Breaking Silence* will likely enhance his reputation considerably. As we said at the outset – we are very, very glad to have read the book." – John Tertullian, *Contra Celsum*

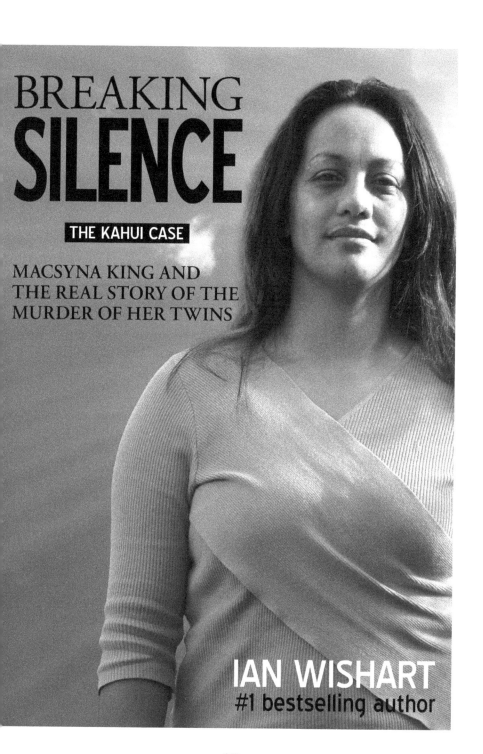

BREAKING
SILENCE

THE KAHUI CASE

MACSYNA KING AND
THE REAL STORY OF THE
MURDER OF HER TWINS

IAN WISHART
#1 bestselling author

THE CRITICS ON *THE INSIDE STORY*:

"Undeniably...when Wishart hits he hits big. *Arthur Allan Thomas: The Inside Story* is a book two generations of New Zealanders have waited for...Wishart...offers an explosive new theory about who pulled the trigger of the gun that killed the Crewes in their Pukekawa farmhouse and theorises about the mystery woman who fed their infant daughter, Rochelle, for days after the murders.

"...With his thorough analysis of the evidence and his generous use of first-person accounts it's a stellar piece of journalism..." – *Southland Times*

"Wishart has a brand new prime suspect and he lays out his case in this fascinating and highly readable book. Wishart is painstaking in his investigation, and his interviews with the man at the centre of the case, Arthur Thomas, offer a remarkable insight into one of New Zealand's most memorable characters. " – Kerre Woodham, Newstalk ZB

"Wishart's report of Detective Sergeant Len Johnston's brazen arrogance collecting items for later use as evidence from Thomas's farm – pieces of wire, .22 shells and axle stubs – exposes a dark and scary side to our guardians.

"Through the book Wishart lays the ground for his claim that Johnston was actually the murderer and by his position on the inquiry team and proximity to Hutton, was able to influence an outcome which saw Thomas convicted twice of a double murder. Wishart's conclusions are disturbingly possible in my view.

"The question of to what extent Hutton had the wool pulled over his eyes by Johnston is moot. Based on Wishart's debunking of transcripts and evidence previously recorded, I think Hutton could well have been fooled by his best mate. Which means so too were the rest of the team deluded." – former Det. Insp. Ross Meurant, *NZ Herald*

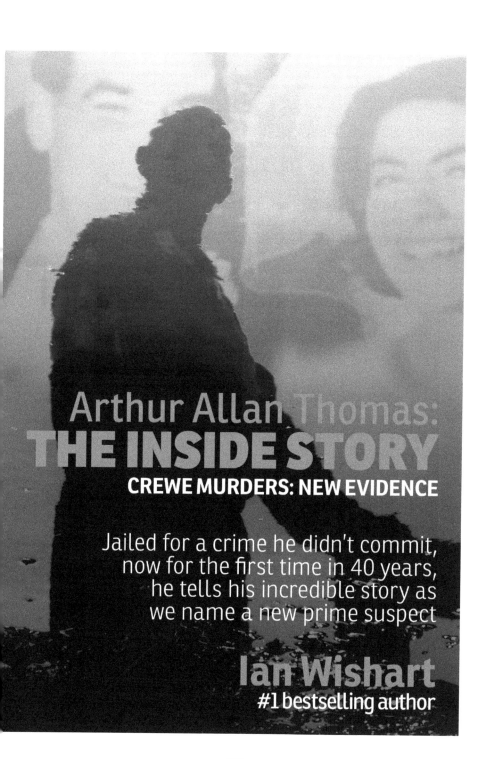

Arthur Allan Thomas:
THE INSIDE STORY

CREWE MURDERS: NEW EVIDENCE

Jailed for a crime he didn't commit,
now for the first time in 40 years,
he tells his incredible story as
we name a new prime suspect

Ian Wishart
#1 bestselling author

THE CRITICS ON *AIR CON*:

"*Air Con* is a thorough summary of the current state of the debate, the science and the politics; it will be an important reference in any AGW skeptic's arsenal." – Vox Day, *WorldNetDaily*

"I started reading this book with an intensely critical eye, expecting that a mere journalist could not possibly cope with the complexities of climate science...[But] The book is brilliant. The best I have seen which deals with the news item side of it as well as the science. He has done a very thorough job and I have no hesitation in unreserved commendation." – Dr Vincent Gray, *UN IPCC expert reviewer*

"Ian Wishart's *Air Con* is another masterpiece of scientific reason, letting the thinking world know that so-called man-made global warming is the greatest scam ever aimed at humanity. Please read this book." – Professor David Bellamy, England

"This book by New Zealand journalist Ian Wishart – a #1 bestselling author four times – surprised me by the completeness with which he reviewed and presents alternatives to the plethora of IPCC inspired spin and publicity which floods our media today.
"His sixteen chapters examining aspects of the debate are meticulously footnoted and thus are a valuable reference resource for those wishing to dig deeper or keep up to speed with the unfolding global warming / carbon reduction political drama in years to come." – Dr Warwick Hughes, climate scientist

"Ian Wishart carefully and painstakingly looks at the topic, examining the evidence and weighing up the pros and cons. He not only finds the science to be unconvincing, but believes that following the proposed remedies will well-nigh bankrupt the West and in fact compound problems. An eye-opening treatment of a controversial issue. – *Quadrant* magazine, Australia

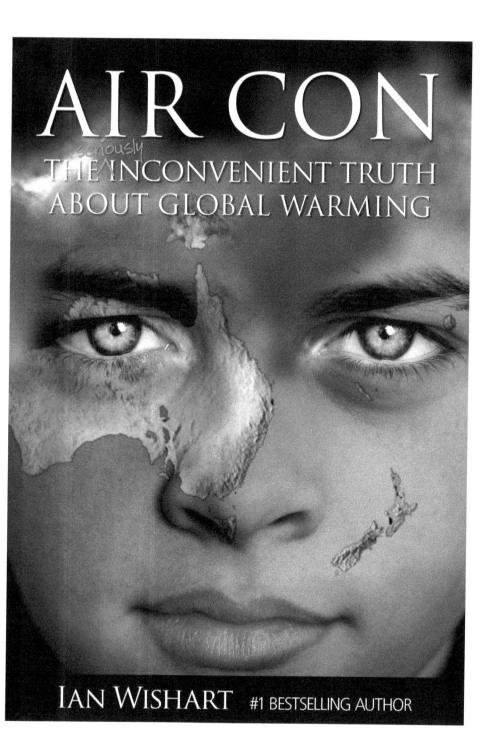

AIR CON

seriously

THE INCONVENIENT TRUTH
ABOUT GLOBAL WARMING

IAN WISHART #1 BESTSELLING AUTHOR

THE CRITICS ON *THE GREAT DIVIDE*:

"Everyone should be reading it"– Doris Mousdale, Newstalk ZB

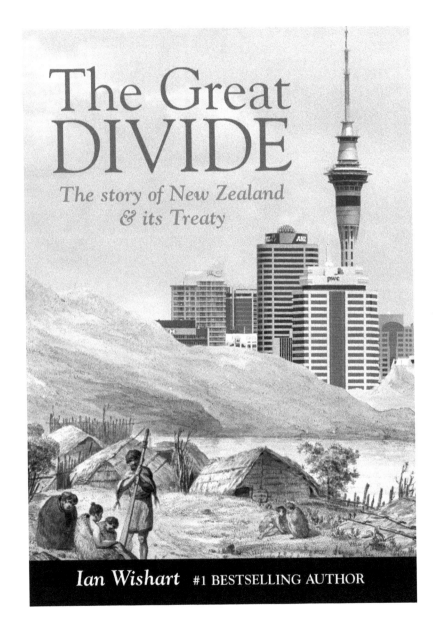

The Great
DIVIDE
The story of New Zealand
& its Treaty

Ian Wishart   #1 BESTSELLING AUTHOR

Lightning Source UK Ltd.
Milton Keynes UK
UKHW021823021221
394974UK00012B/1061